Fucking Law

The search for her sexual ethics

Victoria Brooks

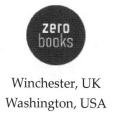

Winchester, UK
Washington, USA

First published by Zero Books, 2019
Zero Books is an imprint of John Hunt Publishing Ltd., No. 3 East St., Alresford,
Hampshire SO24 9EE, UK
office1@jhpbooks.net
www.johnhuntpublishing.com
www.zero-books.net

For distributor details and how to order please visit the 'Ordering' section on our website.

Text copyright: Victoria Brooks 2018

ISBN: 978 1 78904 067 8
978 1 78904 068 5 (ebook)
Library of Congress Control Number: 2018948888

A CIP catalogue record for this book is available from the British Library.

Design: Stuart Davies

UK: Printed and bound by CPI Group (UK) Ltd, Croydon, CR0 4YY
US: Printed and bound by Thomson Shore, 7300 West Joy Road, Dexter, MI 48130

What people are saying about

Fucking Law

For too long, law has been for nobody. Or, to be more precise, law has been for bodies that didn't come as trouble. It is this assumption that Victoria Brooks has tackled in her virtuoso first book, exploring intimately and provocatively what is the most troubling with bodies: their sexuality. In doing so, she has not only proved as irritating as one could be vis-à-vis the certainties of law, but also vis-à-vis the ones of ethics and sexuality. With a little bit of chance, none of them will ever be the same afterwards – for you, as for me.

Laurent de Sutter, author of *Narcocapitalism*

Part memoir, part polemic, *Fucking Law* is an experiment in form which should be read by anyone with more than a passing interest in sexuality, ethics or sexual ethics. Brooks invites her reader to join her in *Fucking Law*, in confronting and questioning the judgments that shape our embodied experiences and knowledges of sex. She argues that we might encounter sexuality otherwise, imagining a new and vivid kindness that would protect our desires from abuse. In searching for an ethics of sex, from university ethics committees to hotel bedrooms to the sands of Southern France, *Fucking Law* offers an unflinching and deeply personal meditation on the messiness of sex, love and philosophy that is at once salty, lucid and moving.

Alex Dymock, lecturer in Criminology and Law, leader of the @ Pharmacosex Project

This book is written by a body, not by a mind: the pages are sweaty flesh, the writing is body fluids, the structure has brittle bones. It is already rare to open a book and feel as if you are looking into a body; but this book does the even rarer and infinitely more generous thing of placing you in the middle of a female sexual explosion. This is a remarkably brave book, relentlessly exposing and yet curing the wounds of the body. This is a remarkably beautiful book, with stunning changes of rhythm and language, but always personal, *ondoyant*, kind, intimate, culminating in a vociferous howl reminiscent of Tennessee Williams's harrowing finales. And finally, this is the book that the law has been waiting for: a book that prises the law open and pours in sex, literary rhythm, corporeal emancipation, female and male desire, French philosophy, and an invigorating full-frontal attack against philosophers. Victoria Brooks is the Anais Nin of the #MeToo generation.

Andreas Philippopoulos-Mihalopoulos, Professor of Law & Theory, The Westminster Law & Theory Lab

Victoria Brooks presents a fierce examination of the relationships between law, ethics, embodiment and spaces of female sexual desire. In doing so, this book offers a bold and scintillating critique of the academy's regulation of sexuality research.

Jon Binnie, Reader in Law, Manchester Metropolitan University

Fucking Law

The search for her sexual ethics

Contents

Preface and Acknowledgments

This book is dedicated to everyone who has been kind to the body that has written it. I think that kindness is the greatest thing a body can do for another body, whatever and whomever it is. Without this kindness, my body would not have been strong enough to write. Kindness is what moves this book, and is the true "Ethics of Her Sexuality" (as the reader will find out, though kindness is not always easy). Kindness is the only way to fuck (with) law. Her story is laid bare here in all its intimate and sometimes traumatic detail. There is no way that she would have the strength to do this without the kindness of the following people:

I thank Andreas Philippopoulos-Mihalopoulos and Oliver Phillips for their love, and who have always been, and always will be, much more than research project supervisors and colleagues. What a glorious journey! Thank you, Jon Binnie, for boundlessly loving this project. Thank you, Júlia Franzoni, for giving me power when it mattered most. Thank you, Oren Ben-Dor. Thank you, David Turner, for Lagavulin Hall, and for never judging. Thank you, Laurent de Sutter, for love and joyous annoyance. Thank you, Lisa Webley, for showing me how to turn kindness into strength. Thank you, Roland Dannreuther, for all the love, grace and kindness in the world. Thank you Danilo Mandic for showing me how to float. Thank you, Wing-Yan Cheung, Matthew Jay, Marc Mason, Martin Cubasch, Simon Flacks, Jack Clayton Thompson, Russell Orr, Eleni Frantziou, Marloes Spreeuw, Tim Sinnamon, each in different ways, for being my lifelines. Mainly, I thank you all for your ridiculous senses of humor and for making me laugh until I cry. Thank you, Ros and Paul Brooks, for your unrelenting support, no matter what.

I thank all my past lovers, for all the kindness you gave. I

1

also thank the readers of this book, for taking the time to read her story, and hopefully, for being moved, amused, confronted, offended, provoked, or perhaps even, aroused...

She fucks law: the beginning of her story

She sat on the sand at sunrise at what was supposed to be the "sexual paradise" of *plage naturiste* in Cap D'Agde, Southern France.[1] Here, the touch of many men, and many women, was available to her. Strangely though, she was longing for the touch of just one man, who was not there with her. She contemplated what on earth she was doing lying on these grains that had captured a hundred thousand free orgasms in their microscopic particles. Her body felt trapped in this "open and free" space. There were three aspects of her identity that she held tightly to her: researcher, lover and woman. In the end, these parts of her mixed together painfully with the sands and waves of the Cap to produce the most *ethical* of encounters. She was at the precipice though of becoming a real "researcher." This is not necessarily what she wanted, nor what she felt she was capable of, since her becoming was going to be difficult. She never considered herself to be an "academic," and all she wanted, all she felt she wanted, lying on those warm, sensual and frightening sands, was the warmth of the hands of her lover, the one man she loved, and to sometimes be left alone to think about things, and stare into space. She had never had much respect for philosophy and its ability to answer any questions about sexuality, particularly her own. It turns out that she was right in this lack of respect. Meaningful insight in fucking comes from fucking, not philosophy: the action, the motion, the feeling, the sense, the provocation, the teasing and taunting, and the breaking of rules. This is the kind of research method she, and perhaps everyone, can understand.

Although others have entered the field of the academic discipline of sex research, she is still alone in challenging ethics (what is right and wrong about encounters) of sexuality *with her own body*.[2] She is alone as a woman challenging the ethics and thresholds of participation in research, asking the very simple question: when is it ethically OK to touch (or not to touch) another body, sexually? This is not a question just for academics to answer, surely. She can only find that thought has not taken the body far enough. The position may be more disturbing than she *thought*. Perhaps the lines we must cross when we reach toward another body are so deep, so resolutely internalized and spread through the blood of the body that they stop the body moving – no matter how radical the philosophy we read and use as our guide. Philosophy has become detached from the bodies that wrote it, and from the bodies that it is written about. We, who are interested in overcoming and agitating these laws, in answering our own questions for our own bodies, must become *fucking* philosophers.

Her hope in allowing herself to be part of this book is to share her stories so that somehow the gap between philosophy and sex might be bridged. Philosophy is tough and obstinate though, since it has grown and been written over thousands of years, since men began to think and forgot to feel. She therefore hopes you will forgive her profanity in saying these laws must be fucked—nothing less will do.

Further, she hopes that her story might empower others to become non-philosophical, pervy, sexy researchers; particularly women, who might contemplate these questions and wonder what they should do where the ethical answers evade and seem impossible to find, and where you might feel scared to even ask. She hopes that her book will provoke bodies to inspect and question the laws which plunge our bodies into sexual quandary. She realizes she cannot answer for everyone, but she does know that others will have asked similar questions, since she knows that sexuality, although individual, is also shared. She knows that her body, although not the same as anyone else's, will have sat shoulder to shoulder with others who have suffered and rejoiced. She always felt privileged to have worked with and had her body fortified and her research strengthened by the voices of many revolutionaries who have also thought about sexuality, and to this she hopes to add her own, even if it is just an orgasmic breath. She wants to show that whatever we have been told is ethical to do (or not do) with our bodies sexually, is up for challenge. This challenge pervades our lives, and it cares not whether we are in the academic field, or in our bedrooms. She advocates the most provocative, insubordinate and playful challenges toward law (the judgments of our lovers, the judgment of ourselves, and the judgments of Ethics Committees and institutions) by the subversive *fucking* power of how it feels to be part of the sexual encounter or event. She calls for the rallying of bodies to join her in an orgy of destruction; the destruction of ethical codes that are not our own, and *fuck (with) them.*

Fuck with them however you can: from behind, from the front, on top, underneath, touching, barely-touching, sniffing, sucking, kissing, watching, gazing, glancing, writhing, suffering, dancing, licking, thinking, loving, hating, sitting-doing-nothing, fucking yourself after watching.

Her story is not told simply for its possible entertainment value, nor its catharsis, although these are excellent side-effects and she secretly hopes for these too. She hopes that her story will erotically excite. Because her story is about sex, or rather about fucking, it would be a ridiculous failure if it did not. She hopes though that these sites of erotic excitement will illuminate too, although sometimes it is just because she feels like arousing you, because she wants to fuck everyone. She tells her story since she is sure that there are sites of glory and sites of suffering, and sites of erotic excitement in odd places, that belong not only to her, but to all of us. Fucking law does not work if she is the only one doing it. Law, and/or indeed our lovers, have a sly way of traversing each of us, and entering every encountering body and becoming part of what we call our *sexuality*. It is our duty, or rather privilege, to fuck with and as part of every-body. It may be the case, as you will read later, that fucking law may only be possible at the transformative space of the beach. But she doubts that, and her secondary hope is that the bravest of researchers, the most titillating and exciting, the most provocative, will find new spaces, ideal for fucking law. Find the most inappropriate, the most ethically challenging, the most terrifying, the most controversial and the seediest; the body philosophy tells you not to fuck.

She lies upon the sand, throughout this book, the potential for an "orgasmic research-ethic." This, as the reader will read, is a manifesto that calls for an authentically ethical research agenda in sex research, but it is also a non-frame for a sexual life: not a code, nor the imposition of a set of rules, but a gentle suggestion of possible questions to ask. Fucking is not so violent and not so profane, not always. This manifesto is primarily a movement: fucking law. Fucking law is a non-philosophical movement which traces and follows sexuality and searches for points of traversal: mutual pathways from mine (or your) sexuality, to that of universal, legal, identifying sexuality.[3] At each point of traversal there may be an ethical challenge to be made, and if this is the case, then we shall make it, and shout as loudly or as softly as we need to, without fear, to ethics committees, universities and lovers alike.

Her book calls for the fucking of law, which the reader will find translates to a call to fuck sexuality, as we see that sexuality really is the *law*, made by a multitude of diverse bodies, from philosophers, to lovers, to books, to institutions, committees, lawyers and judges. She also knows, and has painfully felt, that the sexuality she was told that she had, was not wholly hers, and where it was, it was wrong, and yet she could not find the tools to explain why. She still struggles, which is why fucking is the movement, not the result, and why she needs your help.

Dunes again. Sand dunes. Sand sticks to my legs, burrows between my toes, sticks to my labia gleaming, dripping, fluid stretching in glistening strands between my thighs, a mix of your sperm from when we fucked this morning, and the juice of my pussy. You stand, and with your perfect hands you dust the sand from me. Some of it still persistently clings and rubs as I walk, now and later. You don't realize. Dunes again. Dunes before, a thousand cocks seeking my slit. Then I wanted only one, and now again, the same. Why do these men I love keep taking me to the dunes?

This fucking book

In the coming chapters, she will tell her story. Since she is a reluctant academic, her narrative is, at times, seemingly schizophrenic.[4] She thankfully gives us some coherence and tells us in a more linear fashion the place she came from, the books she has read and the life that led her to become an irritant to her lovers, and to her institution. Because this is all so complicated, and because she knows that such straightforward language and narrative cannot express the power of sexuality, the narrative is consistently interrupted. These interruptions tell us the real, sexy story. The combination of these coherent and non-coherent narratives will develop openings, and sometimes sites of fucking law, which she hopes to create a powerful movement in sex research (whether this be academic or personal inquiry), and in "straight academia."[5] Straight academia is not only the institution, but it is any space where we ask questions about ourselves and our sexuality, and which she has found to be governed by the same restrictions, assumptions and prejudices. Fucking law is the cry of the everyday researcher, every-body, every slippery body that rails against the philosophy and the processes and laws which confuse our bodies into suffering. Sex and sexuality is complicated, but the fucking is simple, playfully and provocatively so.

She hopes that this book will titillate and arouse, in the most bodily of senses, far before and above informing and explaining.

In the next part, she explains what brought her to "research" in this area and she tells you her love stories with philosophers, which took her to the opening moment at *Plage Naturiste*, which she talks about at the very start of this introduction. Although this book is (she hopes) non-philosophical, it cannot be avoided that her research project began as a philosophical one, although she will try to keep academic language to a minimum and restrict her use of overly wordy footnotes, unless she thinks they might be of interest to you. It turns out that philosophy and non-philosophy are predisposed to fold easily into one another, that is, when you think you are simply present at the beach, with not a single philosophical thought in mind, you are following the commands of philosophers, seemingly involuntarily. What is more, reading philosophy can be a rather sexy experience.

Part I

Fucking Philosophy

Chapter 1

Fucking Concepts

Dirty little incomprehensible concepts. Let's be one, together. Breathe their countless consonants out heavily, onto my clitoris. Breathe back in their vowels, violently across the opening of my cunt—IiiiiiiiMMMMMMaaaaahNNNeeeehhhNNNCCCCCSSSSSSssss— the end of immanence felt so almost intolerably delicate on my clitoris, would you do it again? End immanence. I like that fold there, that bit where your shaft becomes your glans, I'll play with it with my tongue, who knew your cock had folds too? You hid them well. I'll lick them with the whole of my volatile body, with my leaking body, my rupturing body, my body that provokes fucking Kant and Hegel and all his friends, and Butler, probably her too, pick any name and tell me their thoughts, repackage them in my image. Tell me what I am, penetrate me, I am a woman, I need to be penetrated, slip inside my slippery slit, destroy me with your words, I can't orgasm otherwise, didn't you know that?

She never stopped being excited by London, where she has lived for over 10 years, since she was 22. Its filthy air and sticky streets and seedy places have always hurt, freed and aroused her, and hurt her again. She loves walking at night the most; when the red-light glistens on the soaked Docklands cobbles, where the faint trace of the pervert's footprint waits for her to place her own shoe within it and wait to bleed out into his body. She likes to experiment, to feel like these men, to be these women, too. She feels like she can, when London gives her this airy and misty gift when she stumbles on the red light, an air which smells of both cosy Dickensian charming domesticity, and the sweat and PVC of the frightening perversion of London's brothels. She is a romantic, and she is a whore. She has been with men to whom she would admit neither of these things, because she knows perfectly well they love and are terrified by both. London suits this perfectly, for her, and has been her most enduring relationship. She thinks about it all the time. She has thought about it since she was a child. She can remember being ten years old and wanting to have sex, although of course she could not tell anyone that, nor did she know about its complex meanings. Her body had yearned for touch, even then. Throughout her life, she has been loved and abused by men. She cannot say she has had a tragic life though. She thinks she has had a glorious life, but people often feel sorry for her; this annoys her, deeply, which means she has become formidable and resilient, yet vulnerable.[6]

On this night, she felt sorry for herself. She sat at a small desk in the room she shared in the house she lived in with her boyfriend for the past five years. When she first came to London, she came because she wanted to be a lawyer; that and she sought the realization of its filthy promises. It turned out that with seeking the practice of law, she found the filth. She came to London and found a flat share, with a live-in landlord, who became her boyfriend of seven years. He was with her through her decision to go to university and become a student at 23. She excelled. Every part a lawyer. Every part a lawyer, since while solving the most intricate of legal problems, she also took cocaine, and went to sex parties and brothels. She did this (she told herself) to please her boyfriend. She suffered, but there was a part of her that did not quite enjoy the experience, but rejoiced in how she could go without judgment, and take satisfaction in the reflections she was brought to feel. The suffering though, is what brought her to wonder if she was the only one in this very strange situation.

She sat at her plain little wooden desk, adding the finishing touches to her final undergraduate dissertation. She had been reading Deleuze and Guattari's *Anti-Oedipus* painfully closely, as if it were a newly discovered biblical text. She wanted it to give her a less painful moral code: a more liberated way of living and loving. Her dissertation supervisor had facilitated her first love affair; she was introduced by him to Deleuze, and after that, he became her postgraduate supervisor, too.[7] The magic of the text was painfully beautiful to her. The text inscribed itself throughout and across her body. It *skinned* her: it replaced a skin, tanned by many luxury holidays, softened by expensive creams, toned by regular exercise and presented and packaged for consumption. The text gave her back her body, and when she looked at it afresh — she saw it as a *Dogon egg* — full of loathsome worms.[8] Her lambent tan was across a taut surface presented to these violent machines — luckily it was slippery as fuck — their grip was clearly not as established as she first thought.

Pornography. I prefer the stories, rather than the images. Stories of men telling me how it feels to be hard. I always write philosophy on my laptop and these stories are constantly there, a fuck whenever I want it during the process of writing, millions of men (and women) waiting for me to succumb to them again. The surge of wetness comes always like a wave:I must stop writing. I have to touch myself, fuck myself, concentration is impossible. Tell me more about your throbbing cock, how you must be touched, how you can't help but fuck. Are you so different from me?

Deleuze ignited in her a fragile bravery. Deleuze ignited in her a rage, but also a sadness. The sadness for her was that her life as it was then had to stop, or rather, it had to *become* something else. She had many rows with her boyfriend. She no longer wanted to be a well-paid lawyer. She turned down offers of prestigious opportunities. She turned down postgraduate study at Oxford. She turned down the possibility of a scholarship at another university. The only path open to her as she saw it, was the only one that was open. It was called a PhD, but all she knew was that she needed some answers, which she foolishly sought. She had no money, and she was told that she would not be supported in her decision. How she loved this new philosophical world, and how it changed her body and gave her a place where she felt unsafely safe, rich with potentials. While her world was turned upside-down, she saw that she could find beauty in the home of other troubled souls. She read every moment that she could. She had never read philosophy before. She was insecure and vulnerable, but she loved these words so much, they touched and caressed her, played with her, without judgment, like no man had ever done.

Deleuze seemed to ooze compersion, like someone sheltering you with their own joy at the possibility they generate for fucking, should you want to. Another of her philosophical fucks in this time, was Michel Houellebecq. She aspired to have the grace of *Platform's* tortured Valerie, or indeed *Atomised's* Annabelle.[9] These female fictional figures she felt were far from misogynistic visions of the Houellebecqian mournful scoundrel, but rather insightfully and delicately sketched visions of a sexuality within her, the trace of what she felt was so misunderstood about her own sexuality. These feminine, motherly, submissive, yet softly strong women, who understood men, and matched their desire. Yes, she loved Houellebecq for this. For this, and for providing her with many orgasms, as she touched herself in the bath, reading his prose. This is not surprising, since Houellebecq is a philosopher too, who took his wife, Marie-Pierre, to the Cap too, to the Cléopâtra libertine club in Cap d'Agde. He took her there for an experiment, or scientific study of social change, or rather, a search for happiness (with a strict and scientific methodology).[10] She would have been interested to talk to Marie-Pierre about her clear penchant for philosophers, and whether she managed to reach the dizzying heights of compersion that Valerie and Annabelle did.

Most recently though, her tastes began to change. Her mind and clitoris are tugged by Preciado's opening to his raging beautiful pharma-fucking, where he cites Derrida's famous line about the questions he would ask, if he could, philosophers such as Hegel, about their sex lives. He said he would expect a very short answer.[11] She found the traditional Houellebecqian protagonist in each of his novels from *Atomised* to *The Possibility of an Island* to be astonishingly astute when it comes to capturing the sexuality of philosophers, and brings a fresh perspective to sexuality.[12]

Sleeping with a prostitute for free. That's not me. Is it? My body doesn't forget your extraordinary beauty like hers would. It will remember you. What do I want you for, anyway? Forever hangs in the sex-soaked air, but why? No, my body will not forget each little hair, each touch, each part of you where the smell is even more intense. Did this prostitute remember your smell? Did she lose herself for days in your memory? Even Houellebecq knows this. Clearly you do not understand me like he does. Don't worry though, they rarely do. But you were the first one to thank me in the morning.

As reader, you will see that the love affairs she had were as passionate as they come. In the mirror, her new body looked different as it merged with her new lovers. Her body was constantly pre-orgasmic, waiting, teased, about to come, the touch constantly withdrawing before she could find the release of orgasmic contraction within her muscles.

Even when she climaxed in the bath, or while she was having sex, the tongue kept on tickling, the words kept on playing with her, the touch running unbearably softly against her surface, again and again, and then she might…but she did not, yet she was open and ready for it: "every cell in my body can open / I have too many / tongues too / many sweet tongues too sweet / for tongues."[13] Deleuze's body of words builds and builds, and then it flashes, and the beauty is inexpressible in its totality, before it washed through her veins, gradually disintegrating into imperceptible tiny fragments of dopamine that eventually vanish into her body ready to be built again, yet forever postponed. This joyous pain! This new masochism she had found!

The dissolved self opens to a series of roles, since it gives rise to an intensity which already comprehends difference in itself, the unequal in itself, and which penetrates all others, across and within multiple bodies. There is always another breath in my breath, another thought in my thought, another possession in what I possess, a thousand things and a thousand beings implicated in my complications…[14]

This erotic power that she felt as she was reading philosophy for the first time can be characterized as the disintegration of her own self, where the body loses its identity and instead becomes one with the text that enters the body. This is not enough for her, though. Stay with her, she is not disappearing into philosophy entirely. This constant teasing is doing her a lot of good. Her hunger is stoked, she wants the flesh of this desire now. She wants to feel how it would be to be allowed to come. To *have* this desire. She can't fuck Deleuze, this is impossible. She can seek someone like him, though. Someone who writes the same magic. She could fuck Martin Heidegger perhaps, like Hannah Arendt did.[15] She did, during her burgeoning "academic career," become intimate with philosophers.[16] It was then that she should have realized that thinking and reading was not enough to fuck philosophy and fucking with philosophy can actually be quite dangerous.

Fucking academia

In academia, as a postgraduate student, it is necessary to go to other universities and tell them about your ideas. Such an occasion is most distressing, for all involved. She felt so out of place among these intellectuals. She knew what she wanted to say, or rather that she had something to say, but she knew not how to say it yet. This time was her first time and the hardest time. She was in the first year of her PhD and she was invited by a philosopher from another University to present a paper. She doubted her true intellectual abilities and potential to have any impact on this world of seemingly frighteningly intelligent men and women, where she was just a bit of a messy whore.

The philosopher who invited her had given a keynote speech

at a conference she attended in her early academic career. She remembered watching him talk. She sat a few rows back from the front and saw him sit there in the center of the room. He spoke like Slavoj Zizek.[17] The rhythm of his voice found its way into her bloodstream, she saw him look at the floor as he sat, seemingly without an audience. He looked toward a corner of the room and he said: "the world worlds, and the earth earths." He paused. What the fuck does that mean? she thought, while her clitoris pulsed. She sat and wondered what it would be like to make love to a man who knew the world like this.

The garden was secret enough, to turn the world inside-out. It was secret enough for a first kiss, that's for sure. After the roof-garden, a secret garden was the only place we could go. We kept on finding gardens. With the bursting into life of each one, all I wanted was to go to the beach, but not the dunes. Never the dunes, but that's where you wanted to go with me, where all these cocks desire me. Why couldn't you just walk with me there, instead of just being desperate to see me fucked again?

For sure, she was besotted with him. A question she was asked at her PhD viva (the oral exam in England following the submission of the written thesis after a period of at least three years) was whether she would do this project again. This was the same as asking would she fall in love with him again, of course she would, in fact, she did: a different man, but he was the same. They always take her to the dunes of the Cap, in one way or another.

She began a passionate affair with her philosopher. She read his work and his big influence: Martin Heidegger. She was told once in a meeting with another academic that Heidegger's texts could never be described as erotic, yet they were to her. She found his penetration into the real depths of her being to be highly arousing, just like her own philosopher. To be sure, the way he did this to her was impressive. She did not realize though that the power was erotic, yet malevolent, violent and outrageously and aggressively unkind.

Her philosopher was married for over 25 years, with three children. They met once in London, before she went to his University to give her paper. They'd had their first kiss within 15 minutes of her arrival and made love that afternoon near a tree in the grounds of the university. They had a romantic, emotional and loving correspondence over the coming months, rich with longing and the need to come together, even if they did not know for what.

Her Philosopher: My life, my moon, tomorrow will be a full moon, repeating itself of the day of our cosmic and earthy kiss, the one that transformed me under the gaze of the quiet passion of the moon, whose light was bestowed on lovers, gifting us. Your hand in mine, your neck, that drowning is the only thing that matters, and which is with me every day, in every tune and sound that I hear, in every smile of people, your beauty that touches every fiber of my being. In you yesterday, I was lost, so much longing and listening again to this song that traces itself so powerfully, again reminding me, again and again, and always that it has not been written, that it cannot be written.

Her: We're all going to die one day aren't we and I don't want to die thinking I lived half a life because of you. I have lost enough time with tears and sickness, anger and frustration and loneliness and jealousy and talking about my sexuality. Enough now.

Her Philosopher: How fucking dare you go to sleep, how can you sleep, let yourself, how can you my love how can you go to sleep? You realize that this is the end of us and you have to let yourself go to sleep, the only way you can escape my judgment.

An intense love for them both led to an intense end. There is depressingly nothing new in this. But what happened in-between for her was the most important of things, for fucking law. When they met, she knew she had to write about philosophy because she had fallen in love with Deleuze and with Houellebecq. She knew too that she had to write about her flesh and her desires, too. But how best to do this, now that she had fallen so deeply in love with an actual philosopher?

She never really knew what "empirical" meant, in fact she isn't sure whether she still does. She knew there was this kind of academic work that researchers do which takes them into the field. It is only now that part of her confusion about this was that she was already *in* the field. But she nonetheless gave it some thought and her supervisors encouraged her to somehow "ground" her work. She liked the idea of going somewhere to watch people have sex in the name of research. What could be more exciting and subversive?

Until this point, she had no idea as to the point of her "project" (in inverted commas since she had no idea what she was doing, she only really thought she had something to say, and studying a PhD seemed to be the only way of doing so). She also liked the company of intelligent men. It was in one meeting with her PhD supervisors that one of them said to her: "why are you doing this?" This was an excellent question, though she found it uncomfortable at the time since she was feeling a bit shy. She knew the answer was that she liked fucking an awful lot, and would rather like to know why this fact seemed so problematic for the world. The real answer should have been this:

Since I was young, far south of the "age of consent," I wanted to have sex with men. Not boys, men. I have repeatedly found myself in trouble, over and over and over again, to the frustration and upset of everyone around me. You are a whore. You must mend your ways. You must settle down. You must do something productive. I have relationships, and the desire is never sated. Never has one man been able to satisfy my desire such that I am able to think of anything other. Then I met my boyfriend, who was as usual 20 years older than me. He said, why don't we have sex with other people together? You can also explore your bisexual side. You can have sex with lots of other men, and I can have sex with lots of other women, yet we can stay with each other. How about that? Yes! Obviously, that's the answer! But I'm jealous. I don't want that. Perhaps I can pretend, and he will change his mind... Why would I write about anything other than what occupies my every waking moment?

She could not say that. In fact, she could not say that until the day of her viva. Instead she said: "I went to *plage naturiste* in Cap D'Agde and I don't know what it is about this place." A boring and rather banal answer it was, but it was good enough for the project to begin. The challenge for her, as we will shortly begin to appreciate, was how to move her thinking from the text to the flesh: from fucking philosophy, to fucking philosophers, from writing to fucking, from thought to movement. How was she going to "think" with her body? While she was fucking?

I suck my fingers. I make them wet, slippery, just two of them, for now. You like this. Licking my pussy juice from my fingers. Juice that penetrates my molecules, and now these fingers of mine smell of my cunt oozings, churned with your pheromones and spunk. My smell penetrates, for sure, I know its power. It penetrates your molecules and finds its way between the hairs of your beard. It dwells in the finest hairs of your masculinity, your chest, that cradles me after we make love and we talk softly and I feel at home. Our smells are mixed: one within the other, within the other. I trace its intensity from your neck to your cock, where my liquid sticks to your sperm and weaves its way stickily through your pubic hair. I just came, but I'm still wet. I still want to fuck. Could I not just turn you over and ease these fingers inside you. I love to watch you squirming, enjoying my penetration, for a change.

A microscopic transsexuality. Just as Deleuze and Guattari had said! But what about the other sexes? Apparently, there are *n* sexes to find: surely here were only two. Surely, she needs to fuck more, to find them.[18] She was also warned by subsequent scholars of Deleuze and Guattari that you have to relax, if you are going to find out more about sex by fucking; you have to be open to shape shifting, from being a woman one second, to a man the next, constantly flowing from pervert to prude, to stable to instable, or otherwise being open to the infinite range of ways there are to fuck and be fucked: *Loving haemosexually does not mean remaining a man, a woman, a pervert, a sex radical; it means opening one's lips to the intensities that flow across a bloody body without organs.*[19]

This strange "haemosexuality" is a kind of BDSM practice which involves the drawing and enjoyment of blood during sex. This was not what she was into, but there was something about this practice which seemed necessary. If she is to see close enough into her own sexuality and to see how it had been inscribed on her body, blood must be spilled, for her body to be open. However, Deleuze also warned of a too precipitous becoming, which creates a suicidal body without organs, a black hole of self-annihilation.[20] A stark warning, indeed. She would need a space that would ensure she felt safe and nurtured if she was going to pursue such a project. She would need a safe space and support, and she would need an understanding lover and a supportive lover.

Sometimes she felt like a man, and sometimes a woman, we know that. Sometimes she felt heterosexual and sometimes she felt like a lesbian, sometimes she felt bisexual. Sometimes she felt chaste, and others she felt like she could not stop fucking. Sometimes she felt like a whore, sometimes a mother, sometimes both at the same time. None of these words could fit her body and her tastes, all the time, but this did not stop philosophy doing its best to contain her, nonetheless.

My philosopher said to me in an email that was a book, after talking to his friend: "after falling in love with you, why is she so interested in this sexuality... coming back to the male issue, she said that there is something in your behavior that makes her worried for me, that there is something quite male in you."

Interestingly, she found that the majority of people who were doing the same sort of work in academia as her, are men. Despite the huge leaps forward driven by feminist thinking, a woman who actively researches (particularly her own) sexuality can be challenging, and at worst, frightening to others. Valerie De Craene, and indeed she, felt troubled by her position as a female researcher in the sexuality field and discomfort at the need to "disclose" her own desires.[21] She apparently "needed" a dose of masculinity before she began her own project. She needed to be called a man, or my sexuality needed to be called male, and her research endeavor needed to be called a leap toward "sexual freedom" and confined to her "male sexuality," to justify it and make people comfortable with it.

Sexuality, *in theory*, has taken huge leaps forward. She was *in theory*, freed to own her identity. But philosophy and its laws are obstinate, since they are not just laws of thought, but they had become laws of the body, too. Post-structural philosophy such as that of Deleuze and Guattari has long since taken the body away from stability, Cartesian separation and Kantian morality, riding on a Spinozan wave to open the possibility for sexuality that is not as "wrong" as she had found.[22] The legal body has been "freed" by philosophy, or so we are told. The legal body has moved from a categorized amalgam of legally owned "parts" toward a body which is as radical as the philosophy which found this to be wrong. Critical legal thought has brought the body closer to a philosophically free body.[23]

Yet, she was starting to hear that people were not entirely comfortable with her wanting to see what it is like to do philosophy while fucking. She had to conclude that indeed philosophy had failed to move away from identifying bodies in such a cumbersome way. She was surprised by the reactions she got from her colleagues, in some cases she was surprised by the support she received, in others she was bitterly disappointed. It would only get worse, when she had to ask for permission from the Ethics Committee at her university if she could go to the Cap as part of her project. Fuck everyone, she said to herself.

She never thought of academia as home. This is not a new thing to be uttered by anyone in academia, though. She did not feel clever enough. Again, a common instantiation of imposter syndrome and relatively banal in some ways. There is something else, though. She had noticed the reactions of her colleagues in academia, when she told them what her research is about. Even with an anodyne version: "I work on law and sexuality"; she saw their eyes change. Particularly the men. She saw their fantasies unfold in their eyes. She was either a lesbian, or a whore. She liked it. She liked to play with this and she also liked to use it as a mode of flirtation, in some cases. In other cases, this was seen as an open invitation to what were unwanted sexual advances and attention, despite protestation. This situation is clearly not without its sadness. Sexuality is a space in which bodies do suffer. Hers has suffered, but others, so much more. The suffering is in marginalization of identities, even punishment in some cases.[24] The suffering is in the unjust representation of sex offenders, and victims, too.[25] The suffering comes from the same place: the insufficiency of judgment to listen to the messiness of the body, or quite simply, to talk about sex in a real way.

So, academia reacts in the same way as the court: discomfort, trivialization and silencing of voices like hers. With the recent emergence of many sexual harassment cases, and in some cases, sexual assault, all kinds of behaviors in different contexts are starting to come under scrutiny. In academia, a whole series of stories is waiting to burst.[26] This is a particularly worrying reality in an environment that has the responsibility of providing an open space of innovation and free discussion which is paradoxically responsible for producing "official" sexual knowledge, and thereby the philosophies that define and ultimately move the sexual body. If we are to properly understand stories of power-based sexual violence and harassment, then the environment needs to be fucked, or otherwise, those who have stories that need to be told, need to feel able and safe to tell them. Academia is resistant to fucking, though. David Bell, for instance, dared to say, "fuck you," and directed a powerful and playful provocation at his field. He found power in the word "fuck" which of course, in most cases will prevent publication or presentation within all but the most radical academic arenas.[27] Bell attributes this fear not only to banal academic conservativism, but a deeper fear of the slipperiness of bodies, such as hers.[28] To say fuck is to ask the other to contemplate the possibility of being fucked: confronted, titillated, rendered unintelligible, perhaps joyous, perhaps destabilized, and at worst, emotionally or physically suffering. Fucking is not necessarily positive, nor is it necessarily negative. The fucking of academia in these times is more necessary than it has ever been if we want to understand the problematic conditions of academia, which she suspects, may well have their root within philosophy, but more on that later. Time for some more fucking.

I could have kissed you for days. Your kiss says nothing about immanence. Your soft skin makes me feel like a man and a woman. Your smell is unusual, not what I am used to. Neither of us penetrate the other, and yet we are fucking. Softly, sensually, sweetly, delicately, increasingly hard. We don't need to be told how to fuck, we just do. I have no idea how long I've been curled in your limbs, how long I have licked you, how long I kissed you. We didn't want anyone else there. They were watching us and our skin was tired by their gaze, and liberated by each other's. All the perversions I have, are fine with you. I can be as slow and lingering as I want. You don't want me to perform. I thought my first time with a woman would render me nervous and clumsy, but it's not true at all. Everything flows just as it should. I really want to bury my swollen clitoris in your folds and rub my soaking vulva against yours until we are more liquid than flesh — I can tell you that, and you don't judge me.

She loved the body without organs. The most beautiful of Deleuze and Guattari's conceptual devices. It could do all kinds of things, but most importantly, it is an irritant within everybody. Just like her, in relation to philosophy. It was her encounters that could explain the power of fucking. She needed to stop loving the body without organs so much though, since this "Deleuzianism" was becoming a machine, too. She needed to turn it into the *fucking* body without organs, if she were to see the end of immanence. She needed to fuck the flesh of philosophy.

You are so English he said. You are not, she said. Radical philosopher and existentialist. You disgust me, with your promiscuity, he said. You are not like my wife, she has something I like in her, like I know and I can feel, that this woman is mine. Mine. You are not like her, not a mother. You are impatient. How could you open your legs for another man? Where is your womb? Womb-an? You are a cold, English, woman. Thank you for last night, said the man who wrote and built my body.

The first time that she went to the Cap was not as part of this research project. The first time was as part of a holiday with her then boyfriend. As we know, she was trying to be part of a "swinging" lifestyle with him, in an effort for them both to have a meaningful and close relationship. This had not gone well, so far. This strategy had already caused her to feel jealous, unloved and caught in an emotionally stunted relationship, where she felt not excited by these occasions, but terrified. She had already managed to be unfaithful, with a work colleague. His desire to take part in group sex seemed to her to have become a way of getting back at her, rather than something to explore together. She nevertheless went, expecting like most occasions for the beach to reflect her experiences of swingers' parties in London.

The red light always signifies the entrance. Not a brothel. The woman at the front desk was beautiful, dressed in her extremely tight latex and stripper heels. She felt dwarfed by this woman's warmth and how at ease she seemed in this most distressing of spaces. She took them on a tour, room by room, bed by rubber-covered bed, by bowl of condoms, by private room, by massive circular bed in the center of the room. The place was dark, lit by a red glow, she nearly tripped in her shoes – she never felt right in high heels. She had her glass of cheap wine. She wished so hard she could be like the other women here who seemed to embrace everything about it. She frankly did not want to watch her boyfriend fuck someone else. She did not want to be watched with another woman, or another man. She was not aroused. Her pussy was shut. She wondered if it was the space, or the man she was with. She thought about it and she was sure she would prefer to be there on her own, perhaps without any men there at all.

The problem was always him. Or rather it was her, with him. She did not want a gang-bang, but she did not want a straightforward heterosexual, heteronormative relationship. She was hungry for experiment and she just wanted to be in-between, she supposed. The swingers club and academia were similar since they were rife with the same demands on her: it was the *assumptions* that were similar, this is what she had discovered so far. Her boyfriend's assumptions (that she would like to be fucked by lots of men, and that this would be a just exchange for his fucking lots of women) were reflected in the institutional fear, or presumption, that this was indeed the case, or otherwise, if it were not, what "terrifying" findings would she unearth? Would she break some kind of bubble or unspoken rule about the truth of philosophy and the sanctity of academia, and its jurisdiction of the production of sexual knowledge?

Her first time at the Cap was before she met her philosopher, so she was not at the precipice of fucking philosophy, yet. She was still deciding whether to dedicate her life to finding answers, or to be a lawyer instead. It goes without saying that she decided on the latter, after her visit.

On your knees, please. Lick me, there. Let me have this. The same saliva that lubricates your mouth, as you say your fine and clever words, your precious concepts, let this mix with the juices you think you understand and in which you seek meaning. I will enjoy this power. My clitoris swells as I watch your tongue.

Chapter 2

Fucking Ethics

She was preoccupied by what is right and what is wrong about her sexual behavior, and preoccupied about why she was preoccupied. She knew she was often told that she had done something "wrong," which generally tended to compel her to do whatever it was again. It caused her to say, "fuck you, I'll do what I want," whether this be directed at her by lovers or by those in authority. On the other hand, she had this peculiar feeling in her stomach, her heart, her blood and particularly her toes, when she did something that hurt somebody else. This feeling caused her to cry; sometimes just a tear that gradually walked down her cheek, sometimes sobs that shook her entire being and made her vomit.

Paul Preciado says that the penis (or indeed the vagina) possesses no more orgasmic power than the toe: orgasmic power is simply the sum of the potential for excitement inherent in each material molecule: "it is the source of transformation of the world in pleasure."[29] She agreed, wholeheartedly; sometimes she came just from thinking of something sexual and squeezing her thighs together, or stroking the inside of her knee, or unbearably gently touching her own breast. But then what of the *ethics* of this feeling. If she could feel pleasure in every single microscopic molecule, then she could feel pain and suffering too. Just as pleasure could reverberate through her, so would the ethics of that pleasure, surely.

It was not a new thing, apparently, to "feel" ethics, or at least to write that ethics could be felt. Spinoza, then Deleuze, then indeed her own supervisor, Andreas Philippopoulos-Mihalopoulos had written that bodies (whatever they may be: a human body, a body of literature, a non-human body, a collective body)[30] have the power to enter encounters and determine together the ethics (what is right and what is wrong *for them* in that encounter). They all "decide" together, in accordance with the responses felt in their bodies. This is not a conscious decision, since Descartes's separation (*cogito ergo sum*) of mind and body had long since been overcome in philosophy. Instead, the consciousness became part of the body and each body, and each part of each body take part in this decision. Decision is better described as "conatus."[31] This conatus is a kind of trigger which prompts the body to respond and move decisively.

This decision, she knew, was not separate from the identity of the body, or laws that judge sexual behaviors. Remember immanence? Yes, we must. We must not forget immanence. We can't, actually. Andreas has repeatedly said there is no "outside." What a ridiculous thing to say, she thought. But wait though. Wait, for fuck's sake. She had always been intolerably impatient. She wanted to understand immediately. She wanted everyone to adore her immediately. She wanted sex immediately. She wanted to feel better immediately. She had not yet learnt to just... slow down.

The problem is that she is suspicious of philosophy and philosophers, as we already know. She has good reason. The problem she now grapples with is whether these seemingly very intelligent expositions of the mechanics of ethics can match with the reality of "conatus." She was sure that Preciado would know more about this than Spinoza, in the context of fucking. From reading Preciado's work, she saw that the warm and exciting *potentia gaudendi* reverberating through each of her molecules, was not without its vulnerabilities. Such a power can be controlled, bought, exploited and, as a result, reinvested into encounters in a way that she was not necessarily comfortable with, in her body.[32] If technology and the pharmaceutical industry could create a "docile" sexual body, which is easily controlled, could not philosophy, or more disturbingly, her lovers, do the same to her own molecules?

With this realization, the ethical complexity becomes infinite, both miniscule and molecular, massive and cosmic. Complicating matters further though is that she cannot turn to philosophy (and indeed philosophers) necessarily, for the answers, since it (and they) have the power to do the same to her body, and the other bodies that she finds herself encountering. Therefore, she had to turn to fucking, rather than sex, rather than sexuality, and this is why she had to turn to law and try to fuck that, rather than philosophical ethics. This is why she must behead herself, behead philosophy, and fuck her way, feel her way, "headless" as she can possibly be.[33]

Where are you now, my philosopher? Did you sit with me and stem my tears, as I wrote this book? As I remember every detail of us? You were happy to fuck me, after you tore my being to shreds, took my sexuality and tried to destroy it and tried to take it for your own by knowing it, at all costs. Remember that one time, after I told you, after months of abuse, after you left me, after you didn't leave her, after you told me about fucking her, that I had tried to make a relationship with another man, but that I couldn't because I still loved you. Remember your silence and your shouting, for hours, your impenetrable wall of words. Remember I turned from you and sobbed on the bed. I was sick with tears. You left me there. You would not speak to me. You grabbed me by the neck and you threw me down — I remember the fury in your eyes — this was not passion, but fury. You walked away from me. I was thin, a mess, in front of a blank hotel mirror. This was one of the last of infinite days of the same. I looked and said, "no more," to myself. No more. There was one other of those days, where instead of leaving in silence, you fucked me over the bath, my nose still blocked with snot, my limbs trembling. Kind of pornographic you said. Obscene for sure. Where are you now? You used the torment of my sexuality to make you come, while you never went and never came to me. The carpet, the purple carpet of that room, the smell of that room and the dried-up mushrooms served for breakfast. Now their deserted molecules sit with

my own, comforting and gently strengthening them, without you.
They join me as microscopic fucking warriors, and no more do we buy
what you said. We sat in our viva, without you. It was extraordinary.
But you didn't leave for long. We fear you are within us. The space
between, that is what interests us now: can we live there?

The practice of law, she thought, was rather familiar to her.
The practice of ethics, perhaps not so much. Fucking law is
what's necessary. There's no point having sex with it, since we
end up with Spinozan ethics, which we have seen are not helping
matters. Preciado's fucking ethic is much more helpful, but she
was not sure about this "headlessness." Law is certainly a bodily
practice; with all the critical legal theory she had heard about
and read, she was left in no doubt about that, *in theory*. It is also
a thinking practice though, too, much to its detriment, so she
had seen, heard and felt. Not much good seems to come of all
the complex logic, concepts and judgments and processes. Law
could protect and come to the rescue of suffering bodies, too.

Fucking practice

She had a suspicion, as we have seen, that law is at the root
of both why conatus cannot be trusted, since law has colonized
the molecules that trigger the body's conatus. She feels that
fucking is so important for changing the way we think about
law's relationship with sexuality. Thankfully, a new wave of
philosophical practice has begun to emerge, but legal practice
however, in the field of sexuality in particular (which is where
one would think it would most likely emerge) is without
radical and adequately fitting versions and visions of research
agenda within institutions. Part II of this book makes a tentative
suggestion as to why, which might have something to do with
the bodies who have the responsibility and control over such
agendas.

The closest vision she found, again in theory, as to the radical
legal practitioner, is the figure imagined by Jamie Murray, a

"critical lawyer." He created the "Vagabond Lawyer" body. For Murray, the "Vagabond Lawyer" is a more sensitive practitioner than the traditional thinking lawyer, able to "explore and intervene" in problems "without precedent."[34] One would assume, as a Deleuzian, that this means a lawyer closer to the bodily-thinking, headless Preciado. But she felt it was not quite this. Although the Vagabond Lawyer is undoubtedly sensitive and reflexive to events, thereby finding "there and then" the ethical balance, there is no mention of the special tools needed in cases concerning sexuality.

Sexuality, as we have seen is concerned with particularities of the sub-atomic, *potentia gaudendi* kind. She felt that these kind of legal problems would need something far more radical than a Vagabond, in order to subvert the investment of philosophy in our orgasmic potential. But she needed to equip herself somehow, with practical tools. She was proposing to move from philosophy, or escape philosophy through the act of researching.

The first time she went to the Cap, was the first time she stood on the same spot as a subsequent fateful sunrise, a year later. She did not go there alone, this first time. This time, she walked with her then lover up along the sands to the east of plage naturiste *from* Marseillan plage. *The casual tourists, families and groups of friends who were bathing in the sun and the sea, began to melt away, the further along the beach she walked. The sun was powerful, even though it was nearly 5pm. She was wearing a bikini she had bought in a small French town slightly north of the town of Agde; she bought it after she had seen a doctor about a urinary tract infection she had and was given antibiotics. It still hurt, but was not as bad as before; it only hurt badly when she went to the toilet. She didn't particularly relish the thought of any kind of sex though and was frankly too tired for all this, and for the impending heaviness of feeling. She stopped dead in her tracks. She looked right ahead, instead of down, at her own footprints in the sand. She narrowed her eyes to try and focus on what was ahead; it looked a bit like a small and sticky Ayres rock. There was this alien-looking mass*

31

up ahead, with smaller masses beside it, spreading from the sand and into the sea. Each mass which was positioned back from the main mass, in ever-increasing closeness, seemed to fragment into naked human bodies, some of them the deepest shade of bronze, some of them white as the purest snow. The main mass rippled in the heat, it breathed as one disgusting body, sweating and slimy with fluid. Against every molecular cry in her body, she kept walking towards it. Soon she was next to it, and it was threatening to overcome her. Thankfully she was wearing that bikini. There were hundreds of naked human beings, and a cluster of them, mostly men, with erections, crowded around two women and two men having sex together. The mass, once she was close to it, seemed to consume every naked body around it, whether they were lying in the sand, or whether they were watching. She could barely find her way through the bodies to a clear patch of sand. The light was an alien Martian twilight color, which made all the bodies look tangerine. She saw legs and cocks and breasts, shaven pussies and men and women of all kinds of sizes. Pumping house music was emanating from the beach bar, making the sand quake beneath her feet. She tried for the water's edge, and was sure she accidently touched people intimately on the way. She stopped eventually beside her lover by the water's edge. She wanted to leave, immediately, but her clitoris was swollen. Her lover said to her that she did not look very happy and she said, well, it's just a bit much, isn't it? He didn't seem to agree, but just looked at her sternly through his Oakley sunglasses, and looked back out to sea, at a group of men, surrounding a lone woman who was tossing off and sucking a random selection of the crowd. She just wanted to go. Very simple. But she came back. And cried herself to sleep, silently, that night.

She did not stop thinking about this encounter, from this moment, to the day of her viva, and she still thinks of it, even now, some five years hence. What took her back there another two times, is the most mysterious of forces: she looks intently inward, realizing she is going to have to do some subatomic fucking. It was her own molecules which stopped her in her tracks at the sight which met her on this day, and the frightening confluence of her lover and those Martian bodies that frightened and teased her molecules on that evening.

This is the problem, you see. That moving from text to field, or moving from lawyer to researcher is a difficult step to take. This means that considering the ethics of practice, and particularly the practice of fucking, as we have seen, is not a banal moral concern, but a matter of life and death in relation to the body. Each and every body has its "lines," that we simply cannot cross. It is not that we should not, but *we cannot*. Equally, we have these lines which we are told we cannot cross, but that *we must*. Some of these lines are common to us all as collective bodies, but it is more likely that the individual lines within bodies will vary. Not everyone, evidently, needed to leave the beach at the Cap on that day she visited, but it is very possible that they might have felt the same as her, at some point, whether they admit it to others (or indeed themselves) or not. These are not conscious lines, but bodily, across all bodies there and then: a reverberation that is felt and causes the assertion of a line, or in some cases, the creation of one.

She read that across the "soul" of everything, these lines are drawn, and in some cases, pre-drawn.[35] It was through recourse to philosophy that she was able to find the possible reasons for the tremors she felt on that day in the Cap. Sometimes the drawing of a line feels so painful that the body is compelled to act urgently. The line on one's soul is not just a cut on an abstract angelic or spiritual romantic entity, but a moment where the body responds by feeling an event physically.[36] Ever had a broken heart? Ever felt so hurt by a person that you feel a cut in your heart, or an ache in the left side of your chest? This is the soul folding. The crack in the soul can be of varying degrees of severity, ranging from a hair-line crack, felt as a "flinch" like a carelessly deployed word, to a full-blown judgment or action against your body, which feels like the ground might open up.

The event could also re-open a previously drawn line and change it from something that makes you cry, to something that makes you dance, or vice versa. The event could turn good fucking into bad, or bad fucking into good;the balance of *potentia gaudendi* is delicate.

She heard the echoes of law here, and the investment of exactly what Preciado was talking about: the creation of the ethics of *potentia gaudendi*. On that day in the Cap, she felt the violence of law's investment into her own orgasmic potential: she was overwhelmed and she felt a line drawn that compelled her to act. Theoretically then, everything was fairly as it should be. She also could find the justification for her slight excitement despite her misgivings, in the "heterotopic" visions of Michel Foucault.

Heterotopia is a concept that tries to explain the existence of spaces like the Cap, by bodies seeking out spaces to perform sexual practices which are outside of the "norm."[37] The Cap could be described as such a space. Great, she thought, it's all explained for her. Except it isn't, is it? Why then, did she keep going back and *not* having sex there, despite knowing she reacted so strongly and negatively toward the space? Why did the bodies look like Martians to her? More than this, what is supposedly "normal" sexual practice? To find these answers, it seemed a seemingly impossible quantum mechanical calculation was demanded of her: she was being asked to split the subatomic and find out, and observe, which parts of *potentia gaudendi* are taken by law, by philosophy and in some cases, by lovers, to be judged and controlled. The demand is increasingly complex and with that, arose its impossibility. To know her body's responses, she needed to feel, express and tell. She needed to say: *fuck your calculation, it is impossible.*

Soul torture. My story, and only my story, is in the smell, and the bed after-fuck. All these molecules play, among the cigarette you think I had at his place. The way my cunt stretched around his cock, and that electricity you think I felt. The voice you think you hear, the orgasmic cries you thought you heard, and the smell you think you own. The enjoyment you think I had. The slut you think I am and need me to be. Each particle you express in your soul-torture carries the specters of a philosopher's oppression and the investment of judgment. Law is spectral in the sex you think I had, but not the fuck. The true ethics, the actual responses of each and every-body, remain invisible, immeasurable and because of that, radical love is never possible, not now.

See, the story told about me is never quite right, she thought. The true sexuality of the moment is never possible to feel, unless you are there. You see, *potentia gaudendi* is impossible to see, impossible to predict and it is guaranteed that your assumptions about its movements will be wrong. It is, like most particles, impossible to measure.

He sends me these photos of his cock. How I love the folds between the skin of his shaft and his tip. I mentioned this before. I also love how he holds his cock in this photograph he sent me. There is this particularly graceful arc of his wrist, and the way his cock perches on his thumb which bends weirdly outward. These hands are other-worldly, there's not much point talking about them, since being touched by them is the only way to know what looking at them does to me. As my eye traces these little folds, I taste the mixture of sperm and my pussy juice, after we had fucked, and all the fucks before, and I smell the air of that particular room, before we went to that particular place, where I never felt so happy. Before you went and I never felt so sad. When you said I shouldn't miss you. How fucking careless of you to misunderstand my body. This image you sent is truly pornographic.

Fucking space
So not a lot apart from minor touching happening on the beach. Now decided to go into the dunes. Walking back into the undergrowth and quickly a large trail of men, of varying ages, stop and then I stop and

I am immediately surrounded by a crowd, touching me, grabbing my breasts, touching me down there, not so gently. I ask for space. A few step back (it's so hot, I feel slightly on edge).

I shout, "Space! Space!"

My cry is echoed by some of the others, who know I will go if I am not heard. So many of them now also shout: "space!" "respect!" I walk now into a shadier part and the same happens, but it is worse, no idea who is touching me now. One asks to kiss me and I say no. I work my way out now, rushing, I am shaken but...is it erotic? Perhaps. I am out. I am out. I sit to have an iced tea and a smoke.

Extract from field diary 14 July 2014 6:15 p.m.

Above is an extract from her Field Diary from when she eventually went to the Cap, taking her notes as the "evidence" for her PhD thesis (she returns to this occasion in full color in the final chapter of this book). This we can see is her attempt to be headless: to hell with any of the rules of faithfulness, and to hell with any of the rules of research. Her cry of "space!" though is rather desperate and it is not metaphorical, but it is a real scream for space, from the deepest innards of her being. It is a cry to have a space away from philosophy telling her what to do: it sent her there, and then left her without the tools to make an ethical decision.

As a lone female in this, what can be characterized as a "swinging space," she is a commodity, rare and prized.[38] It won't be a surprise to know that in a heterosexual "swinging" setting, single women are valued above single men, who tend to outnumber the number of couples, and vastly outnumber the amount of single women.[39] Given that single men are in a sense less valued than couples, and she occupied a space of being valued by both couples and single men of which there were plenty, it is obvious that her body would be *sought after*. She knew this and chose to walk into the dunes, which she had earlier observed as the space where most single men (whether gay or straight) gather to "cruise." It is clear then that she was "voluntarily" exposing herself to a variety of incursions into my space, the reasons for which are highly complex.

She was not surprised to read Ashford's comments that public sex is usually thought of as "gay," meaning that men that partake in such activities, such as at the Cap, or in the practice of "dogging," are "letting the side down,"[40] and not keeping sex private, and their women private. This means that men who engage in these kinds of activities are subsumed within a heteronormative narrative of shame at their "obscene" sexual public expression.[41] Their presence and the presence of sites like the Cap therefore challenges these narratives, posing, as Ashford writes,

a radical recasting of sexuality. It exposes public sex as an activity borne from desire, rather than merely the necessity of historical shaming. Furthermore, if this is an activity in which 'straights' engage, then it raises questions about why public sex is increasingly a point of silence for a gay 'community' that traditionally celebrated public sex as pleasure.[42]

It could be argued that liberal heterosexual public sex practices such as dogging, and swinging, that take place at the Cap raise such a challenge to the shaming of sexual behavior. But this is for men and on behalf of men, but not on behalf of women; indeed she had been left without a guide as to what side *she* would be letting down, or what narratives *she* would be disturbing. The position of the single, lone female is left *theoretically* untouched, but *physically* excessively touched. Of course, it was up to her: she chose to go into the space, or did she?

As Jon Binnie[43] has argued, there is a "soft" quality to queer spaces.[44] They are ephemeral, and they are constituted by and for desire.[45] And as Seideman has argued, queer is not just a space, nor is it a particular sexuality as such, but a politics. He writes that queer theory is a "field of sexual meanings, discourses and practices that are interlaced with social institutions and movements."[46] We find then, that queer theory is that which rubs up against the all-pervasiveness of heteronormativity, or straightness: *Heterosexuality is in some respects, like the air we breathe, a diffuse, all-pervasive presence (a sense of rightness), but, at the same time, out of mind, unnoticed, unrecognizable, often unconscious and immanent to practice or to institutions. The attribution of absence to the pervasive presence of heterosexuality plays a central role in linking certain qualities and values to that subject position.*[47]

This was, of course, the air she was breathing as she entered the dunes. The Cap was not a queer space at all, but a heterosexual one, where she was overwhelmed by the heterosexual expectation. It was within the softness of the queer "experimentation" that she entered the space, the permission that she had given herself, that as a woman she need not be afraid to own her pleasure, as well as consciousness of her superior position as a lone female within the swinging economy. And yet, she was met with the full force of the male gaze, as well as the invasiveness of violent touch. And so, she cried for space, which echoed in the cry of the men who wanted her to feel safe so she would remain and presumably give them pleasure.

What remains absent and challenging to philosophy, and commensurately why it is in urgent need of fucking, is how it feels to live exclusion dressed as sexual liberation. Philosophy as a theory carries the potential to explain and to liberate, as we have seen.

Fucking end immanence

She had heard and seen various references to "intuition." She had been told by her lovers of their "intuition" about her sexuality, their prized "gut feelings" later translated as unbearably spiky and hurtful words. She did not trust it. She also was not completely sure she understood what it is, nor was she sure that her lovers ever understood it either. She wondered if this was the tool she needed to be ready for truly fucked radical legal and philosophical practice. She needed something to allow her to be ethically ready to go to the Cap and step outside of philosophy and of law and set her molecules free.

Preciado's fucking is microscopic, as he undoes every investment in her molecules, even as they are fucking. He sees at once the subversive power of the fuck, because it is there that the possibility arises for a life without suffering, she thought naively, but positively. It is only through such courageous fucking that the investor of the investments, law, can be *somehow* fucked, as hard as that may seem with the constant presence of it in the ethical governance of our bloodstreams.

She sees immanence as the real target here. Beautiful, as it may be. Look at Deleuze's "Immanence: A Life," for some staggering overwhelmingly positive beauty. It's the passage that she always directs her students to: the Dickensian story of the rogue, whose moment of sickness is tended even by those who are sickened by him. This moment of beautiful and positive human purity intervenes as ethical genesis of the kindest form.[48] It is fleeting immanent ethics. It is fine though, for this man, and these people, since here we do not have a philosophical problem regarding the ethics of a *sexual* encounter. It would have been much harder to decide what to do as someone happening upon her in the dunes. What do you do then, with all the complex appropriations from Freud, to Kinsey, to Deleuze, to Lacan, to feminism, to so on to another and another, of sexuality. An automatic response to a dying man is easy, but to a woman in the dunes, it is not.

This for her, is why sexuality is so desperately in need of fucking. Not just connection to encounter, but in trying somehow to float above and feel. Sexual ethics are as complex as they come, because of the lines, both so uniquely individual and dangerously collective. Philosophy is the problem here, resolutely, in creating these lines for us, when really, it is a headless decision.

I was strong and stable. Never again, would I stray. Never, I did not need to. The line is drawn. The big brown eyes, the hands, the same kind of dominance, and the smell, were too much for me. Dive in again. Drink from this seashell, have raw fish at midnight, dwell on these tiny nonsense islands, between spillages of fluids, water, sperm, my juice, saliva, so much kissing we turned to water, words were lost because we were speaking at the bottom of the ocean. You are dangerously exciting, he said to me. The danger, I knew of, didn't need talking about. It was not me who was dangerous, but the fiery philosophies we played with together. It wasn't until that evening, that I fell in love. I think that's why you left so coldly in the morning, because you felt that. That was why I should not have strayed, because, as you said, I should not miss you. But I do. You think my eyes cry with laughter and with tears, and it is my pussy that craves and drips, but it's the other way around. How could you be so wrong?

She searched, long and hard, and it was Francois Laruelle who finally seduced her away from Deleuze and gave her enough courage to step from the page and go to the Cap again. Laruelle seemed to place the onus on this thing called *method*. For those of us undertaking sex research, whether as researcher, or as bodies simply asking questions, doing instead of thinking, is nerve-wracking.

Laruelle's critique of the tools of immanence is that as soon as you utter the word "immanence," you have made a philosophical decision to be caught within it and confined to the (even radical) structures that cannot transcend themselves, simply because they are "immanent."[49] It is making a "decision" to be a woman, or to go to the dunes, or to go to bed with a lover, because you have no other choice. Choice becomes illusory, even among the most radical options, making the possibility of fucking impossible. Immanence might take you to the edge of the page, but it does not take you to the field. It might make you learn how to make love like a Deleuzian, but it is not the actual becoming a hundred thousand between the sheets, or in the dunes.

Ray Brassier critiqued these tools of what Laruelle called

"non-philosophy" as "nebulously expansive."[50] This was hardly a critique, in her eyes. It would first appear that the lack of clarity in Laruelle's definitions would make them unsuitable for her to adopt as a "theoretical frame," yet this is in fact the promise of "headless" philosophy, meaning they were paradoxically, highly compatible. The very fact that it takes a leap from the philosophical to the non, renders such a "non-frame" capable of opening already radical philosophy to its performed (but potentially contradictory) reality. Hickman writes of the ability of Laruelle's work to gently, subtly and surprisingly generate connections with the non-philosophical world,

Laruelle is an acquired taste, not something one can suddenly take up and understand at first sitting, rather one must live with his works and let them resonate off other non-philosophical worlds.[51]

Brassier perhaps did not "live" with Laruelle for long enough, nor was he dealing with the infinitely complex endeavor of splitting the sexual atom. While Laruelle's work is hugely referential, it also tends to take flight from philosophy along a trajectory that has the capability of situating the reader in a uniquely philosophically reflexive, creative and sensitive position that is not inside, nor outside immanence.[52] After reading Laruelle, it is almost like she had forgotten what Deleuze said, yet his words remained etched in her blood (she loved him, remember) and Laruelle reminded her to see how it plays out as we wade in, to see if it works in practice, and then we can decide in the moment, what the ethical answers are, and whether the assumptions are correct, without the inhibiting "crutch" of thought.

This "non-philosophy" although emerging from philosophy, seemed to her to carry the promise of headlessness. She found in his work complete confusion and therefore the possibility of fucking philosophy. She only managed to get here though and read Laruelle because philosophers seemed so terrible at knowing her, yet she found them so erotic. Probably if she met and tried to fuck Laruelle, she would have the same problems as with her philosophers, since this was only headlessness, in theory. You really need to lose your head in sexuality research, but you can't, since the head is ever-so-sexy. The end of immanence is as arousing as the assertion of it, and the impossibility of it ever really ending. She is caught in the middle: a perfect place for fucking.

Now the real challenge faced her. She now had to do it. She had to face all that was to come as a consequence of taking this decision. This was to have a significant impact on both her institutional life, her sex life and the life of her career, in short, her life. It was going to be extraordinary!

Chapter 3

Fucking Methods

We remember what she said about "method"; that she was not altogether enthused by the idea and was not at all sure even of what it is. All she cared about, she thought, was finding answers. But philosophy had taken her, apparently, as far as it could. Reading philosophy, particularly Laruelle, had made her sure that she had to be in the space she had chosen to enter in order to find the answers she sought. Whether she liked it or not, she was trying to write a PhD, and to be allowed to go to the Cap to take her notes, she needed to convince the institution that it was necessary to go there. She also wanted the institution to fund her visit to the Cap (it was very expensive to go there during the high season of July and August). To obtain funding she needed the institution to be convinced as to the "value" of her work. Together with this, she needed to approach the university ethics committee to obtain "ethical approval" for her work. The hardest thing she had to do, and not altogether a separate endeavor to the rest, was that she had to tell her philosopher about her intentions to go to the Cap. Asking her philosopher if he was comfortable with it, and asking the Committee if it would "approve" her project was akin to asking *potentia gaudendi* if the project would pass its mysterious ethical bodily code.

In the end, these questions rest at the core of why she concluded that law was in dire need of fucking, since this really was the nuclear moment, and transformed her project, and indeed her life. It turned out that the question of method is the biggest *ethical* question she could ask: when is it ethical to touch someone?

The Wandering Sands

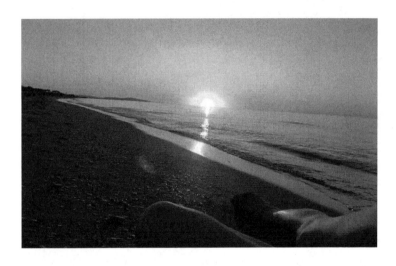

This is the chapter when things get a little technical. But don't worry, it will not last. Also, the photo is important for later, so please do bare with her. This photo is deceptively simple. It is a rather special image, since it was taken by her at the moment of questioning with which she opens the introduction to this book and returns to in Chapter 5. On close inspection, several boundaries or "lines" are apparent. There is a frozen, yet potentially collapsible line between land and sea. There is also a line to be traced along her calf and thigh, which makes her body distinct from the sand and the sea. The effervescent line of the horizon divides the sky from the sea. Finally, the perspective of the photo places her as the observer in the foreground and center, looking out into the distance and toward the rising sun, which also glows upon her body as she lies there on this sand of 100,000 orgasms.[53] These lines are not as solid as they appear, though. The main boundary that seems to collapse, is that between her as researcher, and the beach on which she lies. Coastal boundaries, if they can ever be drawn, do not just leak into the researcher's body, but also rush into, stick to, caress, and cause friction against the skin of her highly permeable researcher body.

This photo, I took for you to share with you where I am. I missed you. I ran down to the sunrise that morning to be near you. Satie, you gave me, playing these pearly piano notes. This man who tried to invade our moment, I sent him away three times. My headphones, my notebook and I, we lay at the start of the world, where the bursting sun made us burst into tears. You told me later how much you hated this photo, and now I know why, it was because you were scared when you saw we were not so different from that sand, after all. I had never seen myself so wet as the next day, as we fucked by email (who does that?!). It wasn't until after a night when, for the first time of many so it came to be, that I sat on the bathroom floor crying at 4 a.m. I was confused why my photo disturbed you.

She had a challenge on her hands. She needed to achieve two seemingly incompatible things: she had to encounter the Cap as free from philosophical instruction as to her identity and sexuality as possible, such that she could challenge sexual assumptions, yet also she needed a method that was going to be acceptable and convincing as part of a philosophical project. In short, she needed something *in the middle*, or something that allowed her to be headless, as well as knowing that the head was a necessary, unavoidable part of sex.

The head is, after all, where the decision to use immanence takes place. But the head does not disappear when no decision is made, and it is not as if fucking is headless. What she took Preciado to mean though is that the head takes no more priority in decision-making (whether it be ethical or indeed methodological) than the toe, or the finger, or the lips, the tongue, the anus or the vagina or penis. Being headless means accepting that the head thinks with the body and not by itself. We cannot cut it off, otherwise why would she have been so titillated by hearing her philosopher talk about Heidegger, or indeed when her philosopher was on his knees licking her clitoris?

She had read about all kinds of methods. Ethnographies, empirical, qualitative, quantitative, interviews, surveys and so on. She had endless conversations about what is best, what the Ethics Committee is most likely to approve and what would be the easiest and least problematic. She read about observing. None of these seemed to fit this question about the ethics of sexuality. How can you answer such a question with a set of statistics? Or by asking a few questions? How can you go to sufficient depth, with sufficient rigor to answer this? The majority of methods, particularly the more scientific, encouraged "objectivity," with a hard line drawn between researcher and field.

Weeks, sometimes months limp by, each day is a long laborious step, as if my bones were made of lead, and my blood of liquid iron, so thick it is from clots of thinking. If you were to dissect me, you would find my brain in my blood. You are coming! My blood jumps and fills my body with thoughts. I was going to talk to you about how hard it is to be away from you and ask you why you don't come more often. It's all forgotten! Instead, each moment has the scent of your neck, the touch of your chest hair among my fingers. By the time we undress each other, you are so hard and I am painfully achingly wet. The longer I am with you, the more the molecules of my body join to yours — I wish they wouldn't — it makes it more painful when you leave. My atoms are devastated, my body a wreck, as yours leaves to be back home with hers, in cooking, laughing, cleaning, talking, everyday conatus. It is not so much that there is a limit to my patience, but a limit to the ability of my particles to recover. The microscopic philosophy is so arduous and so beautiful — our quarks dance together, but mine want to talk about Laruelle, about fucking, about a real life — not philosophy any more. We lay together in this hotel room, one which I had adjusted the lighting in not an hour before, to make it perfect for us. The blank sheets now rich with our sweaty nutmeg fragrance, this room designed for sleeping, for business trips, for tourists, for cheap fucks, is now fucked by our own molecular agenda. I don't know how to start the conversation. We lay in each other's arms. My muscles are tense as my molecules put

their hands over their mouths and mumble muted screams. They say
you must say something. I say: when I go to the Cap for my research,
if I sleep with other people, should I tell you? The balance was tipped:
a silent storm of electrons now, as potentia gaudendi *enters our*
conatus. The smell is even richer than before, as you made a joke of it,
and we began to talk, of you leaving your family for our life together.
Your molecules took their time though, so slowly philosophical as they
are. Such a stupid woman. Did I say what I meant, or was I trying my
best, with what I had, to love you?

It might have been that she was trying to take responsibility
for this extremity of what she proposed to do, and to apologize
for herself. What was clear though, was that method, and more
so participatory method, was a hard thing to do: nobody had
warned her about this. Nobody cautioned her about the effect
on her molecules: the feeling in her toes began to grow. As she
looked to other researchers in her field, she found a bleak picture.
She found Valerie De Craene who found herself in conflict and
discomfort as a woman researcher in geography studies, feeling
a need to account for her own directions, and the commensurate
fear of others of her work, which she bravely continued.[54] She
read Tim Dean's confession at the start of his immersive account
of bareback sex, which assured the reader of his HIV negative
status, to ensure that the reader would not react in violent ways
in a zone of doubt as to whether he was infecting other men.[55] The
point here for her was not whether his project was ethical: this
was his business, and all the better if it were not. Her concern was
the softness of his confession and the strength it must have taken
for him to write those words, and his own personal conflicts in
"choosing" his method (though she doubted that these kindred
spirits of hers had a choice in the traditional sense). She saw
the unrelenting necessity of this kind of work in the eyes of Jon
Binnie, one of her examiners for her viva, that we do not have a
choice, and it is in the name of sexuality, not research, that we
put ourselves through all this. She saw it in Binnie's work too,

and in the work of other courageous geographer ethnographers such as David Bell.

A researcher is living their life, just as any other person navigating the minefield of sexuality. We are all researchers in this sense, or at least this is what she wanted people to realize. Her voice, as a woman, in this sense is alone, painfully alone. With all the strong feminist work, the first fucking attempts by De Craene,[56] the fact that women would ask questions about sexuality with their bodies, as men must too, is still new, and because of that, seemingly devastating for philosophy and all its bodies, whether lovers or institutions. No wonder Preciado wanted to cut the head from philosophy: it is impossible to escape even when we realize the damage of immanence. With the cry of fuck law, comes the shout to other women, she needs you to fuck research as the second level of fucking after philosophy.

This realization though, or this reality, she suspected was not one that academia was comfortable with. It was more than a suspicion in fact, but a harshly felt reality, and this was even before she approached the ethics committee. She only had to read texts on sexuality in academia to find the most resolute turn off. Luckily others had noticed this. Courageous authors have talked about how important it is within sexuality to include one's own story, to add the necessary "juice" to any writing on sexuality. We know how erotic words can be from her encounters with philosophy, so why suddenly, would they become dry?

This is fucking personal

She found that research in the field of sexuality suffers from distance from a sexual life. It tends to be un-sexy, which is not to detract from its usefulness in the field of scientific and empirical enquiry, its rigor, or its importance in its own field. A person's experience of sex is deeply personal, it is the deepest, darkest, lightest, most beautiful and tragic of dimensions of the soul, and yet it suffers the violence of schizophrenic and detached examination, both in method and presentation.

Along with the other pioneers she mentioned above, she found Lambevski's work to be powerfully and unapologetically sexual. Take for instance the opening account of one of his research encounters:

...The tanned polish of his skin, so radiant and delicious, summons the touch of a thousand hands and tongues. His face, so ruggedly sculpted in a few sharp gestures, looks like those rough, yet complete, Michelangelo sketches of beautiful young men. Slightly perched and full-bodied lips meet a perfectly straight nose. His cheeks form two shadowy canyons which allow his nose and deep black eyes to shine in their full glory. His whole face is framed with medium-length, straight, almond hair, thus presenting a sublime gestalt. He shines with subdued contentedness, which makes him almost unbearably sexy...one man after another succumbs to his magic. He cruises for sex with confidence tinged with boyish innocence.[57]

Lambevski proclaims himself an "insider ethnographer," with his overriding aim being that the reader can "feel" the data.[58] Brown's study of homoerotic spaces, specifically public toilets, moves along a similar theoretical trajectory as Lambevski's.[59] Brown's field of enquiry examines the affects of both the material elements of spaces as well as the bodies within them, and how these shape his own experience. He is openly critical of scholarship (particularly in the field of queer theory) which is depersonalised and unsexy, as Binnie suggests: "assimilated into the academy - [such that it] has lost a radical cutting edge. It is rare to find much discussion of pervy sex or bodily fluids. Nowadays you would struggle to find much that is challenging within queer theory - or much to make straights squeamish."[60]

Brown goes on to say that: "...If...descriptions provoke either squeamishness or titillation in my readers, then so be it. The intention here is to reveal the modes of encounter, being and becoming that operate through these spaces."[61] It is here that she sees the extent of her fight. If these men, experienced and accomplished in their field are experiencing these difficulties at the level of text, then what hope does she have in entering the field without suffering? What is extraordinary here though, is her unique opportunity to find the ethics of sexuality, and make pervy researchers of everyone, not only academics. What a gift she has been given!

So be it. Fuck research, fuck academia, fuck law! I will tell you what the law should be, but only as I fuck. The ethics of my pussy are what I bring, the only thing we can all bring, the ethics of our body, our nose, our toes, our fingers, our nipples, our bones, the neurons of our heart (that's where the sensible ones are), the atoms of our blood, the ethics of the pleasures and pains we share, will fuck law from the inside.

The war cry she felt was all well and good, but she still needed to convince academia. She wanted the world to be researchers, but at this point, before she brought her story in the form of this book, she needed to *use* academia, to get herself heard. She needed to give her work weight and authority; she was in the Law School, after all. She knew that the case for the dissolution of the researcher was solid, but she needed a tool, a concept, for making what she proposed coherent to academia.

Others had encountered this need too and found that writers had needed to justify writing their multiple personal worlds into their projects.[62] Fucking law, as we have seen, is a movement at a molecular level, where the slipperiness of the body causes and is subject to quantum cosmic shifts of both individual and universal particles. To be a sexual quantum mechanic requires a view of the world, a path and a tool to help the researcher. It is not so complex, either, and is ideally suited to every-body, or rather to the researchers that we all are in our sexual lives. Fucking law is the constant moving and fucking that is life itself, outside of immanence.

Such a view, or method, is advocated by radical methodologists, Hofsess and Sonenberg. The authors advocate a method which departs (or slips) from traditional research methods and thereby usurps the trap of their assumptions and horizons (or rather, philosophical frames).[63] This in turn allows slippage from assumptions made about the data itself as "stable, knowable, and collectible."[64] During this undertaking, the authors also found themselves reflecting necessarily upon their own presence and how this reveals the inherent "mess" and "flow" of seemingly stable data.

In doing so, the body takes a flight away from its restrictions and assumptions, and becomes a researcher in the most everyday, creative and erotic sense. The secrets held by sexuality, in songs that cannot be written, are only captured in the acceptance that we all have our own experiences and within these the quantum-truth of sexuality is concealed. We can only be near to it, if we live our own and bring it to the world as we write with it and play with it, or otherwise fuck with it.[65]

The Cap

The image at the start of this chapter is no longer of an academic on the sand at the Cap, but a woman who lies on the beach, longing for her lover and asking why she is there and why others are there. These are simple questions with complex answers only in so much as they are bodily, microscopic and constantly colonized by philosophy, and perhaps incapable of being expressed in a traditionally coherent way.

Now that she had decided on how she was going to fool those academics into thinking she was one of them, she is now approaching the time when she must ask for ethical approval (*read: permission to fuck*). This was going to be a fight, she knew it. These laws controlling bodies were important and comforting to a lot of people in academia. As part of this process, she needed to explain and describe to them the environment she would be entering. How ridiculous! How is it possible to describe in a small section of a form, or even in a section of a thesis, such a complex world, her experience of which will depend on everything she has written so far? Look how much she has written in this book just thinking about the space! She is sure though, that you would be fascinated to know what it is like there, so she will indulge your fetish for detail, as she did for the Committee.

She had been to the Cap before, as we know from her encounter with its Martian body. She will now provide for you a "guide" to the space, as best she can, so you can imagine what it might be like to go there and dream about the questions you might ask as a researcher. Like all good tours, she begins with a map (and some helpful facts, since you might want to visit it for yourself...).

The Cap is located to the southeast of the small French city of Beziers and on the west side of a long "spit" of land running from the town of Sète, with the "Naked City" on the shores of *plage naturiste* located at the base of the Cap to the west of Port Ambonne as shown here:

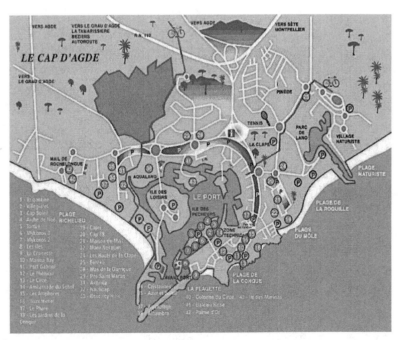

Location of plage naturiste[66]

Zooming further in to the resort itself, the proximity of the "Naked City" is revealed, where most of the nudist and sexual behavior takes place:

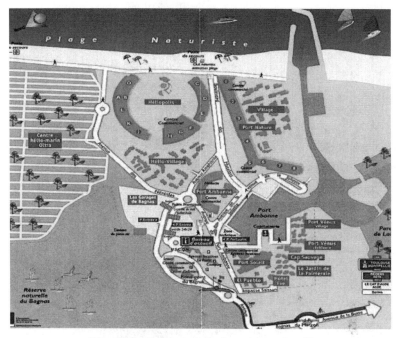

The Naked City and plage naturiste[67]

These maps make it impossible, as a visitor to the space, to discern the locations or type of sexual activity that take place unless you are there. The obscuring of the nature of the space becomes even more obvious, as well as frustrating, when one looks at "Google Street View." The situation does not improve when you virtually enter the resort. You are stopped at the point of entering the beach itself, yet tantalised by a glimpse of the horizon.

It is possible to gain access to the outside of the very apartment in which she stayed (see below) which is the apartment second to the left. It could only be accessed through the gate in the foreground of the photo. This screen capture and the two above look rather alien in contrast to her experience of the space, due to their complete absence of naked human bodies. While she was there in the peak seasons, the pathways and public areas depicted here were usually crammed at all times of day and night with bodies, yet Google has managed to represent a truly naked ghost-town.

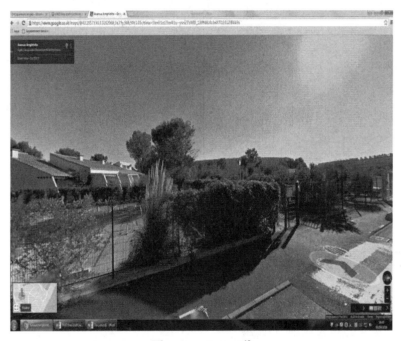

The Apartment[68]

The situation is also similar when one approaches the resort by car. While it is possible to see signs to *"Plage Naturiste"* or the "naturist village," there is nothing to indicate or warn in relation to the kind of sexual activity you may find there. Rather, one is left to discover through word of mouth and reputation of the space. Once you enter the car park, you are unable to go into the resort itself until you pay for either a day or a week pass. At this point, you will also encounter a sign which proclaims *"nudite obligatoire"* and you pass through a gate (she personally found this a rather demanding and disquieting sign when she first encountered it: she almost wanted to keep her clothes on to infringe its rather presumptuous and invasive demand). While there is no enforcement of this flirtatious yet almost sinister rule, it became clear later in her stay at the Cap that indeed nudity *is* sometimes enforced on the beach. It is also possible to access the beach without passing through the official gate and buying a pass; this is by taking a rather long walk from *Marseillan Plage* which is towards Sète to the east of *Plage Naturiste*. Approaching from this side, you will encounter barely noticeable signs which say "nudist beach" as you enter it. You will gradually then encounter an ever-thickening mass of increasingly more tightly packed naked bodies, as we can recall from her story in Chapter 2.

The mapping of the space carries little in the way of traces of sexual activity. Upon researching the space, it is possible to discern that there is indeed a nude beach, on which open sexual activity occurs. Yet the mapping of the space actively obscures the beach from view. On an assessment of the literature, one can gain an impression that the resort boasts a wealth of sex clubs and saunas, as well as a thriving economy, especially during the peak summer months.[69] The "Naked City" (the resort depicted in the above Street View screenshots) is dedicated to the practice of nudism[70] and allows for "free" expressions of sexuality.[71] The resort is located along the coastline, which means it is accompanied by 2km of beach dedicated to the practice of nudism as well as open displays of sexuality, and has a reputation as being the partner-swapping capital of France.[72] Given the high amount of traffic and the multitude of practices which take place at the space, the lack of literature, academic or otherwise, is surprising.

A guide produced by Velton comments that in the mid-1980s the beach itself and surrounding woodland and dunes were used as a site of exhibitionism, voyeurism, and group sexual activity. This behavior continued relatively untroubled by law until the mid-1990s when such behavior was seen to be out of control, since it was taking place in full view of those who did not wish to partake in the scene, or who were on the beach with their families.[73] At this point, the police presence increased to restrict such openly transgressive behavior during the peak summer months (July - early September). Velton writes of the beach that: "police binoculars and horses have put an end to all but the most innocent of contact. In fact, given the often over-zealous enforcement of the hands-off rules by the police, during high season the swingers beach has in many respects become more puritanical than a Sunday School outing."[74] While it seems the presence of the law is felt by those who travel to the beach to engage in sexual activity, nonetheless sexual activity *continues* to take place at certain times of day (late afternoon and early evening) and in certain areas of the beach, such as at the back of the beach, near the dunes, among the crowds and sometimes, in the sea.

D'Onofrio comments on the beach and the emergence of "gatherings" of sexual activity for which it is famous: "scenes with multiple partners, some BDSM and clusters of mildly aroused viewers forming around the most interesting action."[75] She comments that this section of the beach is situated next to an area populated with participants who prefer a desexualized style of nudism, including families.[76] After having set out brief directions which connect with the space and *explicitly* inform the reader what they will find on the beach, she goes on to comment regarding the modus operandi of the space: "all of this is not just tolerated: it's legitimate... Mutual tolerance and relaxed discretion rule."[77]

The sand is so hot I cannot walk barefoot so I need my flip-flops on to set up the beach umbrella to make a base for myself. I am situated on the "libertine section of the beach. **Extract from Field Diary**. *I am sitting directly on the dry sand. I would prefer to be nearer the* *sea but it is so packed that this is impossible without sitting too close to others (or maybe this is my Englishness). Since I put a lot of sun lotion on, the sand is clinging to my skin and I find it difficult to write. Couples of varying ages and a large amount of single men. One directly in front of me as I lay on my stomach on the sand, about 20m away.* **Extract from Field Diary.** *It's nice, the feeling of sun and sand on my skin.* **Extract from Field Diary.** *The thought suddenly occurs to me that there is semen on the sand I lay on. There must be surely. But can't see or feel it.* **Extract from Field Diary.** *Going to walk up a bit, but struggling to remove the sand from my body: damned sun lotion.* **Extract from Field Diary.** *A lot of people (in couples) running across the sand since it is so hot to tread on their way to the sea. This movement makes the flesh wobble nicely...the sand is clinging to me. I think the coldness of the sea would do me some good.* **Extract from Field Diary.** *Several gatherings going on in the dry sand.* **Extract from Field Diary.** *This sand of 100,000 orgasms just allowing me to sit, and how much I desire, just one of those, at the hands of one man. So curious.* **Extract from Field Diary.** *Lying in the sand face-down. The wind is blowing the sand across such that it looks like it is shifting, rising and sinking.* **Extract from Field Diary.** *Sand all over us, in my mouth, I must grab my shawl and wipe my mouth and her breast so I can carry on.* **Extract from Field Diary.** *So I stroke her clit gently (which is also covered in sand).* **Extract from Field Diary.** *So much sand.* **Extract from Field Diary.** *A beautiful sunset, so beautiful, the sea much calmer and the sand is now so cool and soft. So hungry. I miss X.* **Extract from Field Diary** *...many more sandcastles and some impressive sand sculptures at the sea's edge.* **Extract from Field Diary** *...cannot see what from my position which is on the dry sand, but on the edge near the damper sand.* **Extract from Field Diary.** *I sit on the sand watching the sky. It then starts to rain, almost immediately a huge shower, large drops making holes in the sand, I run to the bar and huddle under a straw umbrella with several other people, all talking different languages.* **Extract from Field Diary.**

This flicker of what is really happening is a flicker of the encounters that lay in wait for her in those grains of sand. This is also, as she will find and is expected, at the root of the Ethics Committee's concerns to come. She has her researcher body, she has her method, and now she must seek out what really lies beneath the map by participating with every molecule and story of that space, with every molecule and story of her own. Only then can she carry out her calculations and properly work out what the ethics of her sexuality might be. Brace yourselves, guardians and gatekeepers of fucking.

Part II

Fucking Philosophers

Chapter 4

Fucking Orgasms

The most effective judges of her sexuality have not been Ethics Committees. Not at all. To be frank, she did not care what these anonymous bodies thought of her. To be sure though, they had an opinion. Oh yes. Think about it: it was only by chance that her philosopher was not on the committee. It could so easily have been him sitting there, judging not only her sexuality, but her work, too. In fact, despite his absence, he became it. He became the whole committee and, for a long time, her conscience. He sat on her shoulder, with every man she later became intimate with. He checked what she was doing. He reminded her, with flashbacks of pain, that it would be easier to say nothing. He reminded her that the problem was her, and she spent all her time subsequently, and uselessly, proving him wrong.

She had a taste for a certain "type" of man, this was for sure. The kind of man whose eyes are brown, dark deep wells which mystify and stun her. She is seduced immediately and it feels like this dark grip in her blood. Like every cell is weighed down by wanting, which makes her hands feel empty without holding his cock, and her arms feel useless without gripping his body. She recognized them immediately and could not resist the swelling in her cunt as the scent of them tickled her.

Because of her body's reply to these men, for a long time, she never thought of there being any kind of ethical problem associated with her attraction. She had sex with them. All kinds of men, with "tiger-eyes," eyes that make you think they will eat you for breakfast, that you will be consumed. And yes, she wanted it. She wanted to be consumed, eaten whole. Fucked until she could not stand. Fucked until she could not breathe. Fucked until there was nothing left of her. To be fair, she got what she wanted.

Why can you not find any men you like at these parties? I see loads of women I want to fuck, so it's your fault, for being too picky. She thought about it. It was a fair question. She couldn't think what it was. In the car, on the way to these parties, her knickers were wet. The thought of being fucked by lots of men excited her. Just the little nugget of possibility excited her. That she could lay back and be desired and pleasured. That it was all so very naughty, that she could just have any man she wanted, was delicious. But in her fantasies, the men had no faces. The men had no hands. The reality dissipated her arousal within a second. She pushed at her desire, demanded that it work, shouted and screamed at it to function. But it refused. It stopped dead in her chest, refusing to go south. She sat in darkened rooms, with a glass of wine. Desperately fantasizing to trigger and trick herself into wanting someone. Anyone. She just couldn't do it. She sat with her boyfriend and apologized. She wanted to go home. The truth of it was, that there was no man with tiger-eyes. There was no man there who was cruel enough to dangle love that she could not have before her. There was no man to mistrust her, apart from the man she was with.

Her philosopher met with her in a slightly more coherent state. She at least knew that she was done with sex parties and brothels. The problem perhaps was, that she did not yet know why. It was not until she started to think more carefully about her body, that she realized that there were two massive problems that she alone would not be able to tackle. These problems were intimately and powerfully connected. At the nexus of their connection, she would also find a handy starting point for beginning the infinite task of searching for the ethics of her sexuality.

The first problem was one rather unique to law, and indeed to sexuality, rather like the second. The first is *judgment*, the second is *orgasm*. It is difficult to know which one to begin with, so the only way to do so is to think a bit more about fucking. Orgasm it is then. At this point it is necessary to warn the reader that there will be some masturbation as she tells you about her relationship with orgasm, as is commonly known to be necessary.

Orgasms

She knew several things about orgasms. She knew that she'd had millions of them. From when she was too young to know what they were. She knew also that she'd not had one while having sex with another person until she was 22. She also knew that she would never have an orgasm the first time that she had sex with a person. She was simply too stressed about performing well for that to happen. She was not too sure how she would be judged, so she was better off focusing on the man she was with than on her own pleasure. She could always come by herself, later, if need be. Come to think of it, which orgasms could she remember? The best ones were the surprising ones, where she didn't need to delve into her own fantasies to help her along and she was simply brought to climax by a particular coincidence, where she became space and time, a celestial body, seemingly free of philosophy.

She had just started watching a film on her laptop, having not gone to the beach to do her observations on that day. The night before, she had not slept at all. At 4 a.m., she was sitting in the darkness of her apartment in the naked village, sending heartbroken emails to her philosopher. He had said that he could not stand her being at the Cap and that he was jealous. She sent emails through sickening tears, saying she didn't understand. She was not aroused by the space. Not in the least. They'd had an intensive argument via endless essays during the day. As the storm quietened, and the words began to soften, she felt her arousal grow. The sun was high in the sky and despite the curtains being drawn, the apartment was steaming hot. She could barely breathe. He sent her virtual hugs and kisses, which she felt across her body. Alone, she could play with them, feeling his hands wander from her waist, into her bikini, where her clitoris swelled. The terrace door was open, letting in hot and heavy sea air from the beach and the naked foam parties, all happening in her absence. She was safe from it all. She was wrapped in warmth, intimate with herself. She didn't have to touch anyone, but herself. No one would touch her. But she could watch. She could imagine all that delicious penetration and pretend she didn't care about jealousy and possession. Each atom carried on that breeze gaped open, aching to close around another. Molecular orgies drifted through the door and played with her skin, causing its dermis to morph into the almost painfully red and taut surface of a cock aching to fuck. She wanted to fuck more than ever. The sofa was sticky with sweat, sand and her juice. Her cunt was in that ridiculously wet state, when she felt she cannot continue to exist without something inside her. He sent her messages telling her how aroused he was, describing how he would penetrate her. She wanted to be fucked so badly that she searched for something to penetrate herself with: anything, a deliciously cold cucumber, an erotically shaped shampoo bottle. Penetration was not the only thing though. She needed the weight of a body on top of her. She wanted to open her legs for someone, to lay back and feel like she was being fucked. To feel vulnerable and used, yet safe and powerful, like the opening of her own cunt. From the play of her fingers, she began to feel her orgasm rising in her stomach. It always began there. She felt it like a flavorful yet intensely hot chilli would feel on her tongue: painful yet delicious. The heat would get too much. It would burst out of itself, and in doing so, her whole body felt this heat, like every cell had flip-flopped right then and there in her capillaries. Her breath was withdrawn from her. Her sight was withdrawn and she could hear nothing, not even her own noises. The beautiful sting would twist through every organ, which threatened to burst out of her skin, before there would be, what she thought must be audible, a huge clunk of a contraction in her vagina. Sometimes resulting in a gush of fluid, sometimes not. Then there was this warmth. Like what she imagined heroin must feel like, on its first injection into virgin veins. A honey toasted warmth engulfing her brain, so that she would either fall to sleep, or exist in a daze for the rest of the day. There on that sofa, in the middle of the naked village, she had such an orgasm. She was not sure whether it was her proximity, or her distance, to the fucking on the beach, and to him, that caused its intensity. The following day would be another day of jealousy and judgment, only to grow in intensity toward months and years of the same.

She found the location and time of her orgasms to be insightful. On her own, she could come very easily. In her most lust-filled hazes, she could make herself orgasm in public, without being noticed. She could squeeze her thighs together and have the most intense orgasms within a couple of minutes. She had lost count of the times that she had done so after sex with boyfriends too, when they had gone to sleep after climaxing themselves. When she was with another person though, she sometimes would orgasm just as intensely, but it was rare.

You were full of sleep from an afternoon nap in our hotel room bed, just moments from the beach. A few hours before we had walked in the dunes and had been lying together, fully clothed. It was hot. Too hot to be there, really. I had a thought, while we were there. You knew it too. We sat together in silence among those strange plants that grow in that mountainous sand, looking out towards the sea. As much as you didn't want to say, I didn't want to hear. I didn't want any of it to matter. So I took you by the hand and we suddenly got to our feet. We ran down the dunes and I ran toward the sea. I decided to forget it all as we walked along the beach. I decided to forget that you were another philosopher. By the time we woke together in our bed, I felt close to you, and safe again. You didn't speak, but we kissed, a kiss full of the taste of sleep. Our smells were all over us. Contented fucked molecules all around us. I felt your erection against my thigh. My favorite thing. You barely moved. All I felt was your breath and your muscles flinch in pleasure. I felt the tip of your cock in that between place, just before you enter my pussy completely. I rested there a while, while watching your movements quicken. I fucked you, and it was the softness of feeling the intimacy of our building space, that made me come as intensely as I did that time at the Cap. Even your skin, the surface of your organs, was *soft, despite the hardness. Despite and despite, my orgasm is strong.*

She maddened herself in thinking about her orgasms. She had little to go on in terms of a guide, if she was honest. The books she read would help a little, but conversations with men, or even other women, did not get her any further. She thought that she had orgasms in places and in situations that were not "normal." She thought her fantasies might be somewhat weird, too. It was not until she found Nicholson Baker and his beautiful, intimate yet completely strange *Vox, Fermata* and *House of Holes*[78] that she found playful (completely weird spaceless and timeless) fantasies without jealousy and possession, without tears, and without the violence and boredom of pornography. She was always perfectly happy to watch pornography with her lovers, and sometimes she would watch it herself, when her desire had reached a particularly insatiable peak, and she found herself without a man next to her. But it was a flat orgasm for her. She found play with concepts to not only be intellectually exciting, but erotically thrilling too. What if she turned jealousy inside-out? What if she turned her skin inside-out? What if she played with the boundaries of animal-human, inhuman-human, in her filthy mind? What if she started fucking with paint, with blood, with pine cones? What if, like in the *House of Holes*, she forgot about boundaries, identities, right/wrong, straight/gay, human/inhuman, and instead, did whatever she wanted? What if the world started talking a "new round soft language"?[79]

Because *House of Holes* titillated her so much, she was fascinated. Whenever she read erotic texts, whether Baker's, or Houellebecq's, or Roche's gloriously filthy, stinking *Wetlands*, or even the slightly more serious Réage's *Story of O*, she found the wetness of her pussy to be more visceral than in any other circumstances. It was like when her philosopher was emailing her while she sat on that faux leather sofa at the Cap. The power of this perverse body built by erotic words was such that it touched her with more intensity than a human body. It was crazily pure, without any hang-up, no jealousy, no desperation, no frustrated longing, not even a decision, no waiting, not "oh is this OK"; it was as if she had missed the split second of "consent." She did not need to decide; in fact, she couldn't make a decision. She had no choice whether to be aroused by Lanasha fucking a Magic Kentucky Lime fruit in *House of Holes*, which will give her "extreme cravings for stiff cock" or Shandee's lessons on penis-washing, or her relationship with Dave's disembodied arm, or most importantly, the irresistible Deleuzian beauty of Baker's silver egg hatching, where miniature lovers learn how to kiss and fuck inside a tiny silver egg, forever suspended in ecstasy as they fall asleep in each other's silver arms, wrapped in a wash cloth, destined to forever discover sexuality together. She could not resist Roche's schoolgirl musings of holding cum inside her body for as long as she can, a smelly gift that keeps on giving, oozing out of her pussy, "smiling blissfully in my little puddle of sperm" even while listening to the teacher "going on about philosophical attempts to prove the existence of God."[80]

How familiar that sounds. How touched she was not only erotically, but in a more profound—rather ironically—philosophical way. How futile man's musings are in relation to the existence of God, their attempts to be God through their words, to write the cleverest thing, the rightest thing, and all the while there are these orgasms in places they never imagined. She was convinced that a "soft round language," a language of fucking, was to them, rather trivial.

Good! she thought. Trivial is good. Sexier. More serious. Time: 4:30 p.m. She drew spirals in her field work diary. Round and round and round and round, like a finger, tracing the edge of her nipple, intolerably gently, like the feel of a draping soft and silk cloth, barely touching, then just about barely brushing the pinkness of her nipple. From the outside, the fabric would be tented, a growing nipply tenting. The touch would be so gentle it would cause her skin to erupt in waves, and a hot dull ache in her vulva. The fabric moves to her pussy. The draping is not so successful, since the fabric then sticks, the viscous liquid cooling on withdrawal of the cloth, joyously sticky. Reminiscent of pillows in early mornings and late nights after hot filthy fucking dreams: the cold soft fabric presses desperately against her clitoris. She particularly liked to do this after fucking and being filled with sperm. The smell was so thick, so intimate, so kind, so warm and so safe that she wanted to eat it. She ground her hips into the sand, feeling the walls of her sticky cunt rub together, as she looked right into the eyes of a man at the back of the beach. Grains of soft sand jumped into the wind and blew across her naked buttocks, sand-dashing them gently, like a light spanking, reddening her grinding cheeks. The beach was quiet and she just looked at him, as he lazily stroked his cock. She thought about rows of erections, playing with the idea of touching each one, finding the folds, maybe licking the tips where a small pearl of tasty liquid might gleam. She would touch all different sized cocks, sniff them, taste them, without feeling bad about not making them come. She wanted women too. She did the same with their breasts, she kissed their necks and she walked on her hands and knees, so she could lick the tasty clitorises that she saw. All the while, she stared at the man at the back of the beach. The sun held her back and her sunglasses hid her pre-orgasmic eyes. She looked at him while another man started to suck him off. Fucking, pure and simple: she came just as the sea was creeping up to her toes, between land and sea, between solid and fluid, and with not a thought of philosophy, or philosophers, or for the saltier side of her sexuality. Not despite, but because.

We can see that she comes in all sorts of ways, both associated with, and disassociated with how one might think female human sexuality is imagined, or how (she thinks in her most frustrated moments) the male version of female sexuality is hoped to be. She sometimes likes to watch a woman being taken from behind, sometimes she doesn't. Sometimes she feels like she wants to fuck a whole rugby team, sometimes she wants to spend hours with a woman, just caressing. She likes to play, to think about and to read about, without having to do. She would like to sometimes share her fantasies, sometimes keep them quiet. She wants to feel safely in danger. She sometimes wants the touch of things, rather than people. Of fur, rather than skin. Her sexuality fleets and flits and fucks.

Since Deleuzian thought, the orgasm has been very problematic, since it is the genesis of sexual identity.[81] She feels there is a lot of truth in this position (pardon the pun). Identity, whether it be womanhood or masculinity, straightness or gayness, a big bundle of assumptions in relation to how that person gets their orgasms, comes with it. She never knows what box to tick on those wretched Equal Opportunity Forms that you must fill in when applying for jobs or study. Sometimes she feels straight, sometimes she feels gay, sometimes she feels bisexual, sometimes she feels like a woman, a man, or in-between. She could select "prefer not to say." She always felt that this would indicate some harmful closeted silence about her sexuality though and in fact, evidence pointed to the fact that this would be the most harmful box to tick. She would prefer to say. In the space of those little boxes on the form, she was expected to disclose where and how she got her orgasms and it was categorically not possible for her to tick all the boxes.

You see, the site of her orgasms is part of how her identity is built and the things she is allowed to, or assumed to, desire. This assumption is very important, since it allows the world to know her desire, and therefore, hopefully, tame it and control it, and to stop it causing any problems. Desire cannot be as Deleuze and Guattari had envisaged, as a wave or force that just wants, rather than wants, despite. The vision or image of the space of "despite," or the gap to be filled, is a reflection of outmoded gender politics. It is only through untying sexual desire from pleasure and imaging a future of disruptive gender politics, ranging from eco-politics to the politics of reproduction, that we can give the orgasm back to the body.[82]

The future is well and positively imagined by philosophy.

This is a strengthening thought. But what remains is the question of ethics: what do we do when problems arise? What do we do when our newly imagined and futurist desire, our new and "untied" orgasms cause suffering to something (physical, emotional, psychological), a person, a thing, an animal, a sex robot?[83] In short, when we shed gender, when we shed sexuality and we shed spatial-temporal orgasmic assumptions, with identity fully disrupted, what would be an orgasmic version of ethics? Ought we not understand more about our own sexuality first and find its orgasmic ethic? While the laws of spaces of so-called radical sexuality, such as the Cap, such as libertine clubs and so on are well known, she suggests that the ethics, or that is, the experiences of men and women who fuck there, are not.

The reality of all this is played out at the Cap, with every round of applause with every male orgasm. Male ejaculation is celebrated explicitly, while the female orgasm is less obvious, either in terms of its genuineness, or its genesis. This seemed to match with her unrelenting feeling that identity was never right. This seemed to not be a problem, until it was coupled with judgment. It is the case that judgment gives us our current ethical framework for our desire; that is, that there is (apparently, so she is told) an ethical code associated with sexuality. The philosophical foundations of this (she is told) are solid and true. The philosophers who wrote these foundations are (she is told) very clever, and solid and true. The God who breathed life into these words, knows well both her heart, and her clitoris. Spinoza was a clever man, Deleuze too. Her philosophers. Lots of clever men have written her sexual ethics, so far.

You never told me, but I knew. I would feel her touch on you, as blatantly as I could see the imprints of my feet on the soaked sand. You never told me, but perhaps you thought I knew. I didn't. Or, rather, I did, but only in the abstract. Stupid, I was, wantonly naïve. It took me ten minutes, once I decided to know. Social media can give us away, no matter how careful we are. Within ten minutes, I went from inanely thinking about my day, to contorting with hurt, jealousy, rage and affection on the floor of my apartment. Every swipe of my finger on the screen of my phone brought me another image reporting to me fullness of the potential of the softness I had felt with you in that beach hotel, but with another person. I don't remember when I began to cry, much less when I decided it was not fair to tell you how I felt. What was to be gained from such an exchange, where was the kindness? Yet my heart was broken, anyway. Such a loss. The man I loved was again a married man. Another philosopher. The world seemed to be full of them.

Chapter 5

Fucking Judgment

We then both share her partner's cock, sucking him and licking his balls, she holds my mouth open while he ejaculates into my mouth (and also on my Raybans). Applause. I then get off my knees, exchange pleasantries (as much as I can in broken French and English). So tired. Few men hanging around now, a man (who it turns out is from Leeds, 40s) talks to me. He says, "very sexy," I said "thanks," then eventually ask why he comes to the cap, he says "it's so free, I like to look." The French woman of the couple tells me I suck very well, she said my husband says it's very good. I shrug and say "thanks!"

[extract from Fieldwork Diary]

We have seen that representations (whether legal, philosophical or personal) of encounters and then the judgments that flow can fiercely misrepresent sexuality, by making assumptions about orgasms. She felt that it was neither good, nor bad, to have been part of the encounters that she was part of at the Cap. One thing is for sure though: that she never had an orgasm on the beach at the hands of another person. Nor was she aroused by another's touch. She knew it was not just the sand that stuck to her, preventing the fluids from flowing. When all was said and done, she felt much too alone. While an impressive performance of pornography was clearly appreciated by all who observed and took part either directly or indirectly, it was all rather sad. It could have been the case that it was just her. This was perfectly possible. Maybe every man and woman there was enjoying it far more than her. Maybe their orgasmic ethic was far more adventurous than hers.

But she knew that she was no one special. The space and its bodies gave her so much pain and any orgasm she had was always despite, out of the way, in her dark hidden naked village apartment, or on the sand in her own world. To be frank, she had no idea anymore what was right and what was wrong. It was not only in relation to her philosopher and her philosophy that she felt a sense of responsibility, but also to her own body. How on earth was she supposed to know what to do? She was tired of these questions. She was tired too of the constant questioning that she found herself doing, year after year, hour after tormented hour. She was tired of being alone. She was tired of her own tastes and wished, with all her heart, that she was either one of those brave women who just wanted to have a family and have a calm and kind domestic sexuality, or she was one of these special women who had this "Cap-sexuality," a libertine way of being without jealousy. No matter how hard she tried, she knew that she could never be the woman who lay there watching her partner with another woman. No matter how much the thought aroused her in the privacy of her own masturbation. No matter how much jealousy aroused her in her fantasy world, it destroyed her in its reality.

The thought of her philosophers at home in their intimate worlds without her, and with their wives caused her to spontaneously burst into tears. The sight of dogs and babies would break her heart, since they reminded her of a world she was missing. Yet she sat at the Cap, crying toward the sunrise.

At the beach, ready for sunrise. My my, how wonderful it is and just before simply bursting with life, buzzing in the air, the day to come. All the energy from the night before, the days before and those to come, skulking below the horizon. Reflected in the surface of the sea. It is completely mad here, on my way here, I see to my left, doing some exercises, one of the guys cruising me yesterday. As I knew would happen, on this deserted beach at this time, he starts to run over to me. I tell him I want to be on my own, he asks if he can walk with me, I say thanks but no. I want to be alone, with the sunrise, reflect with some beautiful music X gave to me that he said reminds him of us.

I sit a way up the beach, near to where I was yesterday, just at the moving edge of the sea. 10 mins and the guy comes running up to me, past and then turns back, sits next to me, too close. I explain again I want to be on my own, he says "no speak, just meditation." I nod, but doubtful of this. 2 mins later, he stands up and takes off his shorts and sits back down. I am conscious of this but do not look up, then see him reaching for my foot, erection in hand. I move away and say, "I told you I wanted to be on my own," he says "I just like being near you," and I say "thanks and this is nice, but I want to be on my own," I get up, he asks me not to go but I walk off. I feel a bit bad, but this is my time for myself. I now see a fisherman, calmly walking in and out of the calm sea, just so stunning, magical. Another man with a metal-detector walks up to me and just says "c'est magnifique," I say "oui, oui, c'est magnifique." He walks off. One lone man also walks naked urgently around the beach.

We are the only people there.

Extract from field diary: 15 July 2014, 6:20 a.m.

For her, never were the two poles of her "sexuality" more pronounced than in this moment. Judgment and ways of being judged seemed to come thick and fast at the Cap. Whether it be from her philosopher, or whether it be from the other bodies at the Cap. For her, judgment materialized as a feeling in various parts of her body and at varying intensities. This feeling, she could not escape. Her performance was judged favorably by the bodies at the Cap, or at least they appeared to. She was not judged favorably by her philosopher. She found the assumed time and space of her orgasms to be the foundation of her sexual identity. She also judged, too. She judged bodies as to their attractiveness, and assessed their sexuality (although she tried her best not to). She made judgments about situations and how she should act. These judgments she made were not only intellectual decisions, but bodily decisions, too. The trouble was, that she did not realize that. For all her Deleuzianisms, she still used her head to work out the ethics of situations and did not listen to her body. She thought the problem was with judgment itself, but she realized later, it may well be judgment that saves the day.

"To have done with judgment"[84] is the famous phrase which gives the title to Deleuze's essay in *Essays Critical and Clinical*. Often, she cited this phrase and the essay, as a foundation for the position that judgment is bad. The argument is strong and in some ways, irrefutable. It is hard to disagree with the idea that judgment is at the root of sexual injustice. She did not disagree. She could see that in many respects, she was caught in many courts, where her sexuality would be judged. The problem with judgment is that it is everywhere. It is the very fabric of our structures and it is the bodies with the authority, ability and willingness to judge that glue together the fabric of our lives.

It is well known among philosophers that Deleuze and Guattari were not "into" orgasm, since he had caught on to the idea that orgasm became the site of judgment, as she had seen and felt. Given the complexities of orgasm and the complexities of the bodies which experience its joys and its pains, this position is far too simplistic. Since Deleuze, thinkers have rescued the orgasm, finding it to be the site of infinite creative potential, providing us with opportunities to rethink sexuality outside of identity politics and judgment. She argues though that we also need to rescue judgment, if we are to find a contemporary sexual ethic that works for the complexities of our sexuality. This judgment must not come from philosophy though, from philosophers, or from ethics committees, it must come from the body, amid its dilemmas.

Her body's big dilemma at this point in her search was specifically about the space she was in. With all the sex going on around her, there was a part of her that wanted to push the boundary and to dive into those encounters. She was also sure that she didn't really want to, as we can see from the sites of her orgasms, being technically "outside" of these encounters. But what if it were not a problem with her, or with her philosopher, or with the Cap, but rather the line that law had drawn? What she felt was that the line was too straightforward. Too black and white. Too "you either want this, or you want that."

What if Deleuze was right, that judgments were being hurled at her, as if she were a "void," without the care to try and understand her own knowledge and her own experience of her sexuality?[85] If her philosopher knew for sure how she felt on those sands at the Cap, I mean properly knew, felt and experienced it as if it were his, would his judgment change? Or was it judgment itself, in the hands of philosophers, that kept her and restricted her to her "judged" form? All she knew was that she was on the shore. The shore of the Cap, about to be awash with the surprisingly quick-changing tide. The tide would batter her so much, with the waves so tough and unrelenting in their effort to dismantle her body, that she would be so tired. She would be so tired that she would enter one of those dreamless sleeps, where she would at last escape judgment.[86] But that is no way to live.

Let us examine the tide closely, in the form of correspondence between her and her philosopher, taking place in the few days surrounding the incident of the masturbating Frenchman, the day of the fateful photo on the shores of the Cap, a key piece of evidence, as we shall see. We shall also see the contributions of the Ethics Committee at her university. It will be reassuring to both her philosopher, and the Committee, that their concerns are mutually held.

Judgment: "Handing Down"
Her Philosopher: Just the thought of having sex in public with you can cause me to throw up. So vulgar, so banal, to be

so violent to our intimacy, but maybe there is another side to it, where is the deviance if there is love, so deep and pure. I think that we need to stop for a while. This is what my email said, it was saying that we must pause, stop writing for a while, despite what we feel. Not because of my family and kind of difficulties but because of being with you as your first love. I would feel more comfortable if you were in love before us. You are in love with your love to me.

Her Committee: *The Committee have serious concerns about your safety given that you will be working off-campus with negligible support in a potentially dangerous environment where individuals nearby could be actively seeking a sexual encounter.*

Her: My love, I read over your words again earlier and a chill ran through me that this may have been what you meant. I am lost, I do not now know what to do with myself and tears and tears. I do not understand why the first time I am in love with someone so totally that it makes it precarious, surely there is an element of firstness every time? Cannot sleep, just really in agony, nauseous, it is so hard. I wanted so much the oblivion of dreamless sleep, but I woke after an hour and just the pain, the pain, tore through me. I don't really understand, thoughts of precious moments with you, nearly a year of writing, the longing and the beauty of it, the pain too of course. I get the sense you think I've not been with people I have cared about, which I have, quite a few and some quite long and intense relationships.

Her Philosopher: Don't wait for me, you said that you have become so lonely, I know. You have never given anything to me, never brought anything for me, something material, a thing that I can keep. It was all about us, and how it changed you, so beautiful. It is all simple for you, total and beautiful.

Her: Without its marks? You don't think that there have been days when I have thought to myself that I am foolish to feel this for a man who is just having an affair? Loving you while I know you share a bed with your wife every night? I have felt angry, lonely (perhaps he will take me away, no he doesn't do that, why?). Also, times where I have felt myself like stopping everything, but no, I said to myself he is worth it. Defending our love to friends, who said he will hurt you, he doesn't take it seriously, why don't you see each other more often? And me just saying it's ok, you don't understand, but screaming inside. Wholeness yes, but my lived experience of it, as being "alongside" has not been one of constant beauty and wonder.

I do not think I have ever seen my skin so brown or my eyes so red.

Her Philosopher: I am devastated how it hurts you, but it is not as simple for me as it is for you. I can feel you now, not through your work, not through your PhD. Don't leave me, my love, I want to know you.

Her: My point is that I lost sight of the importance of vulnerability, instead fearing being judged, what will this man, who writes such beautiful words, sends me these beautiful things, whose wife is a dancer, think of me if I opened? What kind of response would I get and I was too scared to find out. Just like I feared the judgment of students, like I feared the judgment of the interview panel. This is hard to admit. Also, it does take time to know me, deeper aspects I mean than my taste in music and film, I have had some very difficult experiences, especially in relationships, some of which I have not told you, but have left me very scared of giving myself, only to be later hurt and left, not just the man that hit me, but other experiences which by email I won't rehearse, unless you want me to, but it would be a long one.

I do admire people who are able to give themselves so easily.

Her Philosopher: How can I not feel that you are experimenting with me?

Her Committee: *The Committee were unclear how you would record the observations, for example would you propose relocating to improve the quality of your observations, and if so how would you be able to guard against suspicions being raised about your activity? Is it possible to undertake covert observations in this way and at the same time remain inconspicuous?*

Her Philosopher: Have you ever felt jealous about me? Have any of your partners slept with others while with you.... a voyeur to your notes I am: "these separate bodies that come together," as you wrote. Perhaps part of the reason was to verify, tease, what you feel towards me... to endure something, what is the stake for you, you feeling the space? Ok you want to take notes for what you write on but the very position of the "note taker" is so interesting, wanted to be touched, not wanting to be touched, where are you in this, as this affective body that moves in the space, naked, not aroused, no, but all of these encounters reminding you of our intimate moments... what are you seeking?

I wrote your story for you, I don't know why: "She is naked, they confess to her, tell her why they come there, and trying to get a fleeting look at her body, at her shaved pussy, bits of sand on it, they can detect some smell of sweat, she is taking her notes. She is so proper and there is something remote and sad about her which is so attractive, so sexy, so free, what brought her here they ask themselves, why does she not want to take part? She needs them to tell her something, too, rather than being just the bodies that she records, something about how she feels. What brought her there is that sexuality that she always felt was so right, so free in her, she came there to see it, she always felt so sexual, that sexuality is there, whenever a man meets a woman, she thought, it is always that question of whether they are going to have sex, how strong it is and beautiful and free when this bodily desire happens, and what and who can stop it, and she wants to record it to see the material environment that people seek for that to happen. Her way of feeling it was meant through this half-restraining herself, even against herself, to record what other people say about it, to resist participation in a way contradicting what she intuitively feels about it, about that very moment of seeing a man that makes her so passionately wet and hot. Sweaty salty chests, hands, cocks, intimacy enhanced by its impossibility.

Her: This isn't me. How much it isn't me. I don't have the words for why, or how, or what I am, but this isn't me. But you can't hear me.

Her Philosopher: I don't leave you, I leave this serene madness. At times, I feel that this just drives me crazy and I don't like it. For a fact, looking now at the photo, I hate it. I HATE it and deleted it. That is what I meant by this tragic aspect, when I looked at the photo today, projected my fears to the future, this nausea, the tragedy to come kind of hit me. I HATE THIS PHOTO and it is so unbearable to hate it.

Her: This is not for email. I do not want you to feel this madness my love, but why on earth would we want to be ambivalent to one another, to not have this intensity? This love for each other that could be so wonderful as it spreads and changes. You are my love, the first time I ever felt that I could just be, to show myself, even felt that I want to have your child at times, that is a strange thing for me to say, but just to feel that.

Her Philosopher: It will be our child, not mine, it will be your child, you will be a mother. This is so beautiful that you feel for having my child. How can all this be, so quickly.... it is so beautiful and yet so frightening to me. It is so trivial and funny and so banal and cheap really, somebody looks at supreme beauty and masturbates at your sight, and funny in a silly way, and insignificant. But look what it did to me, this distastefulness, suddenly everything in this photo looks cheap to me, and I know how you felt and I do not want to hurt you but this is how I feel, it's over with this photo for me. What did you think it would do to me, you just told me an anecdote about your curious experiences at that moment, and you being this object of wanking while being with me, simple on the cool sand with Satie right? Fuck!

Her: What I say about feeling like I could have your child, it is about the oneness I feel I suppose instinctively, and yes, I know it is quick to say it, to seem to be feeling something like this, so quickly and intensely, but there is madness there for me too, about us, how I feel about you.

Actually, I am glad that you are done with the photo, that it has come to disgust you in this way, because I hate it too. I hated it there. I hated your reactions and I hated how alone you made me feel. This photo represents bad memories.

Her Philosopher: You are so adapting to change...just move on....and then....and then...."I am actually glad that you are done with the photo"....oh. You still don't hear me. Well you do.... there was nothing wrong with this photo. Anyway.... tired of that really....

Her Committee: *Concepts of privacy could be contentious. While* *the research will be undertaken on a public beach, the individuals being observed may view their area as being a private or semi-private space. As there are quite strict laws in France relating to privacy has there been any assessment of the legality of the proposed research in the local context? Can you confirm that any proposed covert observations will only take place on people who are in a space that could be reasonably observed by others, the individuals would have no expectation of privacy and that you will not follow individuals to better observe them should they go behind bushes/ into caves, etc.?*

Her Philosopher: Stop being banal. Everybody projects... but not everything is projection my love. Reactions speak for themselves in word and in deed, in judgment.

Post-Judgment

Judgment. The possibility of it, as well as the aftermath, made her anxious.

It was not an overt and obvious state of anxiety, but a constant state of being on edge, when she feared judgment, couldn't leave because she knew it was wrong. She appealed so many times, eventually exhausting her right, when she was clear that no matter how much she tried, the judgment would not be overturned. However much evidence she submitted, however much she dreamed of justice and woke from repeated dreamless sleeps, the judgment was resolute, tough and immovable.

She felt stupid and frustrated with herself. She'd had the benefit of so many sources to help her with her search for sexual ethics, but all she ended up doing was fucking law; none of these sources warned against this danger! Perhaps it was unfair to make such a demand and she needed to take more responsibility for what happened. There is no point in all this, unless she can come up with a new way of judging the ethics of a situation. Because she suffered, and he suffered, both then, and after she returned from the Cap, she found that it was even more important that she share her findings with the world.

To have done with orgasmic judgment

The main source of her suffering was that she had nothing on her side. Judgment was against her, which was inevitable. Even her own body was pitched against her. It transpires that judgment will rescue her and so will ethics. These two rather conservative philosophical terms will renew her body, and will be something she desires to share with everyone else, particularly those who find themselves in the situation where their sexuality, or indeed their love and kindness, or their naivety, or their desire, or lack of desire, their desire for love, or their simple presence, is abused. This abuse might not only occur at the hands of other bodies, but also by law too. Law, both legal and philosophical, is the source of identity, and the power given to judgment vests in these, through the power it gives to bodies ill-equipped to be gentle and kind.

Not every judgment will be a "bad" one though, just as not every law is "bad." But as relates to sexuality and love, she has no fear of saying that every single law and judgment is bad. Rotten to its very core. It is only through changing the very function, movement and result of judgment, restoring to it a core of kindness, that we can find the ethics of sexuality. Looking back at the above judgment, we can find why she can be so sure that law's relationship with sexuality must end, before we move on to look at how she thinks we can become newly and properly sexually ethical, through a new, persistently flexible and bodily sensitive way of judging.

Judgment and Ethics (institutional)

We can see from above that the Ethics Committee was concerned about her safety at the Cap, and also that they were concerned that she keep an inconspicuous distance as Note-taker, as well as ensuring that her project would not cause the onset of privacy litigation, should "participants" discover her.

Already we see the Committee resorting to all they can: judgment. The first judgment is about her gender. Straight away, they know she is a woman. The second judgment is about her vulnerability because of this. The subsequent judgments are infinite, when it comes to her sexuality. As many other researchers have found, the participatory female sex researcher is an "incoherent" body. They do not get the same benefits as men, in the form of the "veil of professional silence." This means that while male researchers might have sex with their subjects in the field, there is an "understanding" that this happens, but it will not be talked about.[87] Certainly in the 90s, it remained "outrageous" for a woman to not only have (or indeed not have) attractions during her fieldwork, but even more scandalous were she to write about these attractions. The context that women researchers operate in is one that is anxious about the apparent "incoherence" of female sexuality and is in a rush to attribute such a sexuality to being a sex radical, or worse, deviant. The reality is of course that pushing against identity, particularly sexual identity for women, is hard work. It is important work too, not that this is acknowledged by institutions who would prefer masculine distanced work, which ignores the realities and context of the field. Institutions prefer quantitative work, or the kind of work that will yield funding, and present as an attractive research agenda for research councils and students alike.

The odd reality is that work that pushes against the boundaries is now, in the current context of the fierce momentum of feminism and anti-establishment politics, of great value. This does not appear to be the case with sexuality work though, or rather it is, unless the work speaks dirty and uncomfortable truths about the bodies of institutions, both academic and philosophical, and their role in the persistent structural injustices done to female sexuality.

The Ethics Committee did their best for her. But the problem was that they were caught within the law, meaning their "best" was not good enough. They had to consider the legal concept of duty of care and intimately connect this with their judgments about my gender and sexuality, while operating in the context of the neoliberal self-interested, erotophobic and sex-backward institution. While they were doing this, they had their own bodies to contend with. We sometimes forget that ethics committees are comprised of real human bodies, with their own sexualities, and of course, their own prejudices. It was perhaps somewhat lucky that she had some supportive bodies around her, and in that Committee, so her ethics application was eventually accepted. But what if she did not? What if this was not the case? In "risky" sexuality work such as hers, will other researchers have the same "luck"? We can see then that law and judgment open this space for luck of the draw, which simply will not do. It cannot be the case that the ethics of a project in participatory sex are based on a judgment on legal principles. This must stop.

There were three of them, which she hand-selected, in the end. It was a slow night, at the only night at the libertine club where single men (men without a woman accompanying them, as a couple) were allowed. She was not particularly interested in fucking any of them. She did it to please her lover at the time. She willed arousal in herself, but with nothing. Luckily, it is hard to tell. The slipperiness of the gross lubricant covering the latex of their condoms meant that no one noticed. She felt numb, actually. She didn't feel bad, or forced, or anything like that. But she felt bored, and tired. It was hard work. One of the men, a tall American muscular man, with a frankly enormous cock, was her favorite. He had a kind smile and was very gentle with her. He was the only one she kissed and had on top of her. The others she cannot even remember: their faces, their cocks, their movements, nothing. She drew a blank, entirely. What would someone think, seeing her there? She was knackered afterwards: her body ached through and through from all the positions and contortions and the countless demands of three cocks. They all agreed — unanimous — that she performed well. When she left, she felt nothing, really. Only that she would find it impossible to tell this story, without sounding like a whore.

Judgment and Ethics (her philosopher)

She was justified in her concerns. The reader will remember some things about her philosopher. He was married. He was also, he said, in love with her and thinking about how and whether to leave his family, for her, at the time of her leaving to do her research at the Cap. We know that he was scared (we don't blame him) and we also know that he decided she was "experimenting" with her monogamous side (for this, we do blame him). All in all, though, it was a difficult and ultimately abusive relationship and to be sure, she did things too that she was not proud of. There is one reason though that she cannot and will not take ethical responsibility for the abuse that she received. This reason is philosophy.

The extracts above represent a tiny fraction of an exchange that took place across a two-year period of around 10,000 emails, thousands of text messages, heated phone exchanges (one where she threw the phone across the room in frustration, only to pick it up again, and he was still talking, without noticing any interruption), and many long meetings. Many of these times and exchanges were wonderful, loving, full of humor, and were some of the best times of her life. But many of them were the very worst, when she didn't think there was another way to be. She has still not shaken his ghost, which haunts her in the form of crushed confidence, even as she writes her story. Thanks to the kindness of those in her life, she has found that she has reconstituted as a much stronger, kinder and happier body because of her experiences.

She went into the relationship with her philosopher not knowing the rules. She too was preoccupied by law and judgment. Some, perhaps the ethics committee, perhaps others, would suggest that she had been unfaithful, and therefore deserved what she got. There were many moments when she thought so too. But she would stop herself. This sexuality that her philosopher gave her, was not hers. She was told that she was not a woman. That her sexuality was wrong, because it was not womanly. So therefore she had to be a whore and frankly, her philosopher was relieved. He even said to her, of one of her open confessions to him about her sexual encounters that he liked her letter to him, since it showed him that she was not for him. She was not the kind of woman that he could love. It was far from a coincidence that we hear strong echoes of the concerns of the Ethics Committee here.

It did not matter what she did, in the end. The ethics of the situation were not that she was in a relationship with him and therefore she must be faithful, nor were they that he was married and so therefore she was able to do what she wanted. The ethics of the situation were that when it hurt, it was wrong. Her responsibility was only to understand *why* it hurt, and for that endeavor, philosophy was totally useless. Law too, was totally useless. How would it help her? Would the judges come and be able to see through the laws and philosophies? It did not matter to the Ethics Committee, either. The aftermath and the suffering were far outside of their contemplations and their visions of risk, which in the risk assessment was limited to whether she would get sunburn and drink enough water. There was not talk of sex, nor really, properly, risky sexual encounters, nor the emotional isolation and vulnerability that can come from such a project.

Law, as we can see, has no use here, whatsoever. She did not want the law to tell her who was right and who was wrong, or who should be punished. She did not need the law to tell her to apply sun block, to sit beneath a parasol in the direct sun, and to ensure she hydrated regularly. She didn't want to apply the consent framework for the Sexual Offences Act 2003, or the rules relating to emotional abuse in relationships: her philosopher did not cause a breach of the University's ethical code, nor their duty of care. It was painfully obvious that none of these laws would help her and none of those would help others, either. Nor would the liberal philosophies of jurisprudence, not Bentham, nor Raz, nor Hegel and not Foucault and not Deleuze. In short no philosophy written by a philosopher would help anyone. No philosophical debate, no moralistic exchange and no extensive correspondence would result in finding her sexual ethic. No code of research ethics, nor any instruction manual would help us find the answers.

Philosophy is as old as life. Would there be life without philosophy, or philosophy without life, you asked me as we shared a bath. I don't know what you're talking about, I said. The first time we fucked I was on my period and there was blood everywhere. That was a bad omen. I remember being embarrassed, but you didn't care. Didn't care that I was embarrassed. You told me you love me on that first time. Another bad omen. Apparently, you told me later, that I was cold when I did not say it back and when I dressed too quickly to leave. Leaving. Leaving hotel room after hotel room after hotel room, in varying states of brokenness. This means that now I cannot be left in hotel rooms by anyone, without crying. Those kinds of spaces are scarred forever; perhaps they always were though, before your legacy. I am still good at finding them. The philosophy changes. It hits a different register, more honest, in a way. The next body tells me more about his authority and prowess, before the next and the next. Tell me, philosophers, which philosophy applies to my sexuality? You filled me with your concepts earlier, while we were fucking, and now they are stuck: our soul-child is conceived. I'm not scared of judgment: the thought of fucking to conceive is erotic as hell. Perhaps you were right, sadly. There is no philosophy without life.

Chapter 6

Fucking Kindness (to have done with philosophers)

She often heard the word "kindness" mentioned in the same sentence as the Cap. The impression created was one of erotic benevolence, where the environment was free of "judgment." To be sure, it was the case that a man could masturbate and be the voyeur wherever he wanted on that stretch of beach, even if he was not invited to touch and be involved. From what she saw at the Cap, this was true. It was as if every man there was like Bruno from Houellebecq's *Atomised*, who felt the overwhelming and rather emotional benevolence of young women who let him watch them, as he ejaculated uncontrollably on the sand. She couldn't deny the presence of *something* soft and giving at the Cap, which outright refused to find sexuality to be threatening and in need of control and judgment. The feeling had a melancholy about it though, too. It was a soft melancholy, that seemed to accept the decline of desire and be soft and gentle toward it in its time and space of inevitable decline. This soft melancholy can be found too in Houellebecq's prose, as each and every male protagonist in every novel fails in his search for happiness. She failed too, as we have seen very clearly. Might it be though, that they, and indeed he, and indeed she, was too quick to reject judgment?

It was true too that she had often heard the beach described as a sexual environment where women were in control and their desire should always be respected, and their word would be final. Indeed, she never saw a single encounter where a woman was openly forced to do anything and just a small gesture, or even a look, would be enough for a refusal. Each man would, without fail, keep his distance, until invited to participate further. That being said, she could not account for the number of people who, like her, would have orgasmed only in private, or had experienced the same ambivalence that she did. Maybe there were none, and every single body that was there, wanted to be there. She had her doubts.

She was at one of these foam party things, a club with a pool, which was immediately behind the beach at the Cap. It was very blue. The floor was blue, the pool was blue and the toilets and shower rooms were blue. Surrounding the place were high boards, topped with Perspex, so the whole place was like a bubble. This was presumably so it was not possible to look inside from the rest of the naked village. The place was crowded with naked people, which is not surprising since upon entry it was an absolute condition that everyone must be naked. This already did not put her in a good mood. Who did they think they were to insist that she remove her clothes? She didn't have to let anyone see her naked, surely. She walked nervously around, this time with her boyfriend. He seemed perfectly happy. She thought maybe a drink would help, so she downed a glass of terrible wine. It made her feel hotter, and more removed. How come everyone else was finding this so easy? She sat with her boyfriend by the pool a while and looked at what was happening. A black woman was swimming in the pool, occasionally stopping to talk and flirt playfully with different men. She watched her with envy. She wondered if these men were ones she knew, or ones she'd had sex with at the Cap, or ones she had just met there and then. She jumped in their arms occasionally and smiled and laughed. She wished she was her. Instead, she sat there nervously, probably miserable looking, at the end of a sun lounger. She wanted to talk to this woman and know her secrets; perhaps she had the key. She walked with her boyfriend to sit on the edge of one of these plastic bed things that surrounded the pool, designed for group sex. Her boyfriend was anxious to have sex with other women than her, a truth that hurt her daily. She thought, if only we would, then we could forget all this, for a while at least, and instead go on normal holidays to the Greek Islands or Venice, or perhaps even the rest of the South of France. She thought she must just do it, and then it would be finished. It was just like porn, she reassured herself. No love, just fucking, no need to be jealous. No need to be hurt. It's all in front of you to see, so there can't be any harm in it. There's no cheating. No unethical behavior, what is there to worry about? She repeated this mantra in her mind, over and over. Her and her boyfriend sat next to each other on the edge of that plastic bed. It was not long before the woman from the pool was sitting on the opposite end of the bed. She was talking to a female friend of hers and presumably her lover, and another man. They seemed a happy foursome, talking, laughing and smiling. At some point, the woman from the pool started kissing one of the men, and then sat back down and was sucking his cock. The other woman did the same, and quite soon, the two women were on all fours, next to each other, being fucked from behind. It was clear to her that there was an invitation to her and her boyfriend to join in. It was clear not only from the occasional glances, but also the small crevice of space which was currently dividing them, was crying out to be filled by their bodies. She could not move, though. She just watched. Her boyfriend leaned towards them. She was confused. In the privacy of her bed, she would often masturbate to the thought of her boyfriend fucking other women. Beautiful women with perfect soft and tight pussies. The more he was enjoying it in her imagination, the harder she came. But here, where the potential was actual, she froze. Her desire was frozen too. She desired nothing other than walking away. She felt sick, she felt sad, and she felt jealous, and she felt affronted and angry, and she felt alone. She saw her boyfriend, erect and ready to fuck these women, and for her to be fucked by these men, but she was feeling the opposite. She wondered should she just sit and let it all happen. But she can't, she'd be expected to do something, otherwise she would be ruining the mood. She just stood up, said to her boyfriend that she had to go and she just wasn't feeling up to it. He was, understandably, she thought at the time, frustrated and angry with her.

It seemed to her that desire often contradicted itself. The amount of times she felt frustrated with herself, at her lack of bravery and her lack of erotic generosity, were infinite and painful. She wondered if it was time to give up on desire. Or maybe it was time to accept that she was simply very conventional and not worthy of an adventurous desiring life, filled with erotic adventure. She was not Valerie and she was not Annabelle. She may have been like Marie-Pierre though, but it is impossible to know. What was for sure, though, was that if she followed philosophy, and indeed the word of her philosopher, she ought to have been Valerie and Annabelle. It occurred to her that this might have been the reason for the melancholic feeling at the Cap. Perhaps it was all these Valeries and Annabelles that had managed to fulfil their potentials and fit Houellebecq's vision, but at a cost to the space.

Fast forward some time. To a different time and a different space, far away. She was in bed with a different man. He could so easily have been a philosopher, eager to know everything and apply the appropriate laws and give the correct judgment in accordance. She was curled up with him in a warmth that she had never known before now. They watched films together and cooked. He is strong, masculine and kind. He listened to her nervously tell the story of the foam party, with a shaking small voice. After she told him, she was scared that he would no longer be kind to her. But he just said that it was a sad story, and that she was just trying what she could to be loved. It didn't matter to him. He called her a pervert and made love to her, he listened to her fantasies without flinching, without demanding their actualization. She was surprised at how the Cap lost its power, and how judgment can free someone, as well as harm them. She was surprised too at time, and how she could feel it in the changing conditions of her body much more clearly than she could watch it pass. She was surprised too at how far from complications, morality and sexuality ethics were, and how obvious the answers were. The fucking was amazing, perverse, ethical; she never found herself so wet, and so often.

It is possible that we can reduce her questions to the simple division between fantasy and reality, and the difference between good and bad men. But we all know that it is far from as simple as this, as the distinction between both dichotomies is far from being clear. We know from Deleuze and Guattari that the actual is immanent within the virtual; its future feeds and unfurls with the present. With every fantasy, the further we are brought to questioning how this would be to actually experience. Yet we are limited in the performance of our fantasies by what is legal, what will pass the conditions of judgment, and what will pass the conditions of ethical codes laid before us. It is clear though, from what we have seen in her story, that such a framework does not function ethically.

The Cap is a place for the performance of fantasies, and as the law will confirm, and indeed philosophy will confirm, there is nothing wrong in that. There is nothing to judge. It is not only your clothes that you will leave at the gates of the naked village, but your judgments too. She wonders though if it would be better to keep judgment, just in case. It was only after her experiences at the Cap and at the end of her project that she realized she needed to urgently restore judgment, in some form or another, when it comes to sexuality. The fact that all the sex at the Cap was legal, permitted and indeed encouraged by philosophy and by philosophers, that made her sure that law's relationship with sexuality was doomed. The melancholy in the air and the degradation of the Naked Village as a sad utopia, made her sure of this.

As she has said, there were no blatantly non-consensual sexual encounters at the Cap. The correspondence of the Ethics Committee was in defence of her personal safety. The correspondence from her philosopher was also in defence of love, of himself, and of the Cap, too. Everything on the face of it was right, ethical and legal. But her body screamed otherwise and she wonders whether the stories of others would be similar. Not all of them, but some of them might shed some light. This is where, at last, she lays the foundation for a renewed judgment and a renewed search for the ethics of her sexuality.

We know about the sources of the problem and we know how terrible law and philosophy are. We know there are lots of philosophers out there, too. So, what do we do now? What of this search for her sexual ethics? It is all very well to say that judgment must end, that enough is enough, and that judgment must be reborn, re-formed in a more sexually sympathetic way, but how will this look? How will we judge in this new way?

About time

We find ourselves now in a unique period for sexual ethics. In the wake of the #MeToo movement and the strengthening of the feminist movement, we have seen structural inequality become the target. With this being the case, the bodies who have responsibility for these inequalities have also become the targets. It is those in power who now have the uncomfortable yet necessary task to reflect on not only their professional relationships, but their sexual ones too. It is with caution that this movement must proceed, as the backlash to the necessary feminist movement has been a radical misogyny. If we look to the disturbing internet space of the "incels" ("involuntarily celibate" men),[88] we find men speaking out on forums, who have fully shut down in response to feminism, and found themselves radically entitled to women's bodies. It is easy to categorize this backlash as simply that: backlash, new, reactionary, repulsive, or almost justified as a marginalized position. It cannot however be minimized as a movement, nor reduced to a few stupid people who are simply monstrous. To do so would be to cover the real sites of masculine vulnerability (which is a serious concern given the apparent suicide risk) but also to risk not going far enough with the urgent reflection and sustainable structural change that the renewed power of feminism calls for.

It is with significant discomfort that she reflects on her own sexuality, her tastes and her experiences before, after and during her time at the Cap. It is also with resolve that she realizes the true destructive power of philosophy, and some of the bodies who crafted, spoke and wrote it. In these final sections of her book, she makes her case for the renewal of judgment through a non-gendered, yet highly erotic, movement of kindness. The most non-judgmental kind of fucking law, and for searching her sexual ethics.

To have done with philosophers?

She found it an arousing question to ask herself. Would these men who are so clever fuck in a different way to the ones who weren't philosophers? Would their touch be different, would sex be something out of this world? She also wondered when this weird fetish would finish; would it make a difference once she felt more empowered? Or was it rather that she had a fetish for concepts? Was it philosophy she wanted to fuck, rather than the bodies of philosophers? But then, as we know, we cannot separate the two. Turns out that yes, philosophers do fuck differently. Beautifully, in some cases, extraordinary, in others. They were not all the same. The ones that held too tightly to their concepts, took them too seriously and talked incessantly, not letting her sleep and not letting her dream, these were the ones who sometimes went from extraordinary to painful, in a blink. From wet to dry, from open to shut, from pre-orgasmic to a very flat post-orgasmic. At such times, there was no soft honey enveloping her brain, no playful conversation and resting upon his chest, no sniffing, no kissing, no sharing food, no sleep, no gentle soothing licking of her clitoris, no laughing. There was only the big problem that philosophy had with the orgasm, that it was the end of everything and time for a bad and complicated kind of judgment. All she could do was wait for it to pass, while she listened in horror to the way her sexuality had been written and how it was to continue to be written.

As we know, it is not possible to unravel the body for the concept it thinks and writes. For that reason, we can always see philosophy and philosophers as one and the same. We also know that in some cases, the orgasm is the big problem, since it becomes the site of a problematic kind of sexual judgment and identity locus. Her own sexuality found arousal in all kinds of things, despite and because of her attraction to the difficult figures of Houellebecqian philosopher men, and in all kinds of complex ways. It is not as though these men were at "fault" in any way, and nor was she. She is not interested in assigning blame. What she objects to here is the power and authority that these kinds of bodies can have over the construction of sexuality. This is a big deal.

It could be the case that she too is responsible for constructing an identity. This may well be the case and it too, like her identity, has its erotic power for her. The problem is far deeper than this. With life comes philosophy, and for centuries, millennia, men have grappled with finding their place in the world. With the intellectual power of philosophical thought, comes the power to control the body. Remember how much philosophy has turned against its own separation of body and mind? How much it has moved from inside/outside, to fractal continuum? How far it has moved from categorization not only of mind/body, male/female, alive/dead, human/inhuman? How true it is that philosophy has made huge leaps and extended its reach like never before. Everything has become a concept, and thus falls within the possibility of being known by philosophers. Philosophers have never been so powerful.

The writing of philosophers in clever books, peer-reviewed articles and endless conference presentations and key-note speeches has been subject to constant checks through peer-review, criticism and lively and fierce debate, both in person and online. Yet the effects of the bodies of philosophers and their sexual power, has not. This is usually silenced. The power of the "veil of professional silence" is far reaching, even though everyone is fucking each other and there may well be a thousand stories like hers. This reality can easily be cast aside as a "personal" life, with no professional or institutional consequences, but this, she suggests, is a dangerous game to play.

Silence on these matters can be erotic and it can be fun and playful. This she does not criticize nor seek to prevent (indeed she is not one to talk, for her story with philosophers continues). Speaking on these matters can also be problematic, for its possibility of breeding a new kind of surveillance, and this is something she resolutely and violently objects to. Rather, she suggests that in this age of the need to know everything, that we do not let the privilege of philosophy, and philosophers, extend too far into sexuality, since their judgments are more than likely to be wrong. Not only might these judgments be wrong, but the privilege of philosophers might mean they are able to write rules that are wrong, and which might feed into institutions with the power to shape the way we "do" and "think" sexual ethics. After all, what did all these men, from Plato and Aristotle, to Spinoza, to Deleuze and Derrida, Heidegger (especially him), Hegel and Marx, to Goodrich and Zizek, know about her fucking sexuality? How do they know what is important to know, what it is important to do, what it is important to say, about her fucking?

In finding her ethics of sexuality, she finds it is important that she realizes that not only bodies and philosophy are part of sex, but concepts too, in the form of bodies. Concepts are powerful things which can control bodies: they can excite and titillate, they can give orgasms, but they can also control the movements of bodies, stop them from doing what they want, make them do things that are not good for them, and make them suffer too. They can be ignorant too. Sexuality is one of the worst concepts—it alienates everyone and everything, even orgasms—meaning we find our bodies abused. Sexuality itself and concepts of identity must not be strengthened in this ethical search; they must be treated like we treat every other body in our sexual lives.

To have done with philosophy

Thankfully, we have seen from the work of Preciado that it is about time we started to be careful with pharmaceuticals, just as we must be careful with pornography. We must be careful since these things have the power to invest our bodies with agendas that are not ours, or otherwise turn us into docile and compliant bodies. The attacks come from all angles, even as nano-warriors in the bloodstreams feeding the very minds that create the concepts she seeks to disempower. Laurent de Sutter painted beautifully the malignant anaesthetic power of philosophy (despite being a fucking philosopher himself; *interesting, she thinks*), as well as the persistent resistant power of the fucking body (and the fucking mind).[89] A fucking body never shuts up, never backs down, and never gives up, despite the equal and opposite philosophical and pharmaceutical force that invests and reinvests the body in directions that are bound to numb it; even the womb is not immune.[90] Philosophy will again and again reassert itself and its prowess and power over her body, through the conflicts and endless contemplations she finds herself during her search, and the endless "despites" and "becauses" of each and every orgasm.

You see, with every ethical dilemma, it is inevitable that one starts to think philosophically. This is a trap. One starts to think, what would other women do in this situation? What would men do in this situation? What is right according to morality, justice, and beneficence? What is legal? How will I be judged? What should I do despite, or because of these things? The time and space of my orgasm should be this, so this is my identity, and my ethical code accompanies this determination. What does the law say on this point: it says that I should/should not be suffering, so therefore this is my answer. The philosophers and the judges say this is right and this is wrong. The philosopher and the judges are only bodies like her, and like you and me. Although they have an undeniable authority over the body, this does not mean they know the orgasms of each and every body. Since law has been built by philosophy (and vice versa), both are places we should avoid when searching for sexual ethics.

You never know when right and wrong is going to hit you. It is never written down and never fixed, a bit like my orgasms. I think it is somewhere in the dunes, back in July 2014. Or was it every time I felt my whole body was in a knot, scared of you, but I don't know why, waiting for the next email, sick, looking at my laptop. Was it when we fucked over the bath, or was it later, nearly three years later, with a man that treats me kindly. Was it when I saw that couple who were naked on the beach, clearly in love, completely lost in each other and oblivious, uncaring about the bodies around them, arousing in me great jealousy. When I went into the dunes that time, I felt brave. I felt sure that the ethics committee was wrong and that fucking was all that mattered. Aroused from a lack of fucking any real bodies, I paced and prowled the dunes at 3 p.m.,the very hottest part of the day. Fuck you, risk assessment. No sunscreen, no clothes, no fear. I was sweating and horny; the sand seemed to have the same footprints as the cobbled streets of London. Steps of brave perverts before me that I was retracing. I saw the overspill of waiting men between the dunes at their opening. I was scared to go in, but I had to. Every part of my body had become the concepts I wrote and I had heard said about me, each of them persuading me that I wanted to fuck. My clitoris said yes too, this thing succumbs easily to words. I took a breath and turned left into the dunes. Gazes of the waiting men followed me as I entered. There was not a single woman, or couple, back there. When I was behind the dunes, the whole landscape was dry and arid, with these strange sand plants and trees. I saw men in all directions, either standing or sitting stroking their cocks. There were far more than I expected. The sun was so bright and hot that everything looked fluorescent and skins glowed and shone. I was hit by a sudden awkwardness; what do I do now? I panicked a little and turned right. I walked slowly and carefully, not wanting to trip. I looked behind and there was a group of about ten men gradually following me, all walking and stroking their cocks. By the time I turned back around, there were three men in front of me, forming a block in my path. I carried on. I then realized, that since this was the dunes, my path was suddenly blocked: this was a dead end, and there was no escape. I carried on as far as I could and thought a gap in the bushes might allow me out into the main beach. The way was too narrow and the bushes were prickly, not wide enough for me to get through. I had to turn around. By now, there were nearly twenty men behind me. I thought they would probably keep their distance. I was wrong. I tried to walk back through. I had no sense of whether I was aroused or not any more—I was simply scared, but I was still determined not to be beaten—my arousal will beat yours! My feminine desire is more powerful than yours! I'll show all of you, even you philosophers out there. I stood completely still and faced the crowd. One man stepped forward and touched my breast. Then another. Another man got on his knees and started to lick me. I did nothing. I have always considered myself a passionate and affectionate lover, but here, now, I did nothing. More and more men began to touch me. Something within me gave up. I wanted to get out, but I couldn't. I became the center of that Martian body of heaving sticky humans. I lay still and saw myself from above. The only time I protested was when one of the men tried to kiss me. Otherwise, I let it all happen; hands too rough on my vulva, tongues all over my body, clumsy grabbing of my breasts. Sperm started to coat my skin, from all those men climaxing on me. In the center of that body it was hot and humid, filled with groans and swiftly moving knuckles along desperate and lonely, or hot and horny, or confused and hurt shafts. As the bodies began to dissipate post-orgasm, I saw from the ground a couple approaching slowly, holding hands walking through the dunes. They kept approaching me. She had long black curly hair that almost swamped her body, and the reddest lips. Her skin was pale, so they could not have been at the Cap for long. She sat on the sand beside me and offered me some of her water, from which I took a small sip with a shaking hand. She helped me up and we talked in a small way in broken English and German. She asked me if I was alright and took my hand and led me away from the dunes. By now the sun was kinder, as was the sand. She looked at me, and suddenly, we ran together, into the sea. I never run into the sea, since it is usually too cold for me. But I ran like never before. I grabbed at the waves like I was going to eat them after months of starvation. I dived into them. I never dive. I washed myself in sea water and released the dead sperm that was coating my skin into the waves. I closed my eyes tightly and let myself sink. I jumped back up, remembering the kindness of that woman, who really did nothing and everything. I found her floating on her back, and we swam back to shore together. We sat on the sand, with her partner, and we had ice-cream from one of the over-priced sellers that pace those sands, sneaking a look at the bodies lying naked and fucking. We didn't fuck, they didn't ask. As I walked back, I kind of wanted to, though, and felt the tiniest pang of regret, and wetness between her thighs, she came thinking about the touch of that woman's skin, and her long black hair tickling her breasts, by herself, on her last night at the Cap.

The ethics committee would probably have imploded at the sight of all of this. Judgments would have been flying all over the place! Philosophy would have a field-day! Frankly, when all is said and done, and all analysis is over, when judgment (in the traditional sense) is over, and we have looked at her path and how it brought her there, once we have undertaken the required psychoanalysis, all that mattered was her need to get out of the dunes. Whether she wanted to be coated in the sperm of strangers unconsciously or not, and the morality or immorality of this position, is irrelevant to the fact that she needed to be away. This is also irrelevant to the fact that the woman led her away from the dunes and treated her with kindness. These two facts have no root whatsoever in philosophy. They are resistant to analysis and, she would suggest, are the only ethics that matter, and the only ethics fit for her sexuality: fucking sexy ones. Sexy as hell.

We have seen in through the popular (albeit still complex and mind-bending) theoretical physics of Carlo Rovelli that we must accept the possibility that time belongs to consciousness and our limited human perception and philosophies.[91] Time is events and bodily states, with no real difference between past and future, aside from the heating up of molecules. There is no "flowing" of time, and no romantic river, through which we flow — forever can be an eternity, or it can be one second — as those who visit the Cap, or anything like it, will know. She would like to take further Rovelli's moving conclusion (though she is no scientist), that time is merely an instrument. Rovelli tells us that time, as philosophy, and thought, and our human compulsion to order, is our way of "handling a substance that is made of fire and ice: something that we experience as living and burning emotions. They propel us and they drag us back, and we cloak them with fine words. They compel us to act... Sometimes it is a cry of pain. Sometimes it is a song... [the song] *is* time."[92]

Fucking is time. It is that very fire and ice, the elemental and molecular activity of our very existence, that makes us feel alive and connected (in boundless love and boundless pain) which we try our best to order, through philosophy. For this, she cannot fault philosophy, or indeed philosophers, since how else do we come to terms with what we believe to be the passing of time, the passage from pre to post-orgasmic. How else do we make sense of it all? It is interesting that Rovelli finds that it is the "song" rather than the passing of linear time that compels us to act. Rovelli is a philosopher though, so we must be careful. His conclusions are no doubt beautiful, moving, and mind-expanding. The critique of philosophy is that it contains time and this too has been the criticism of philosophy's relationship with space. Rovelli is a philosopher too, just like Newton, Aristotle, Einstein, Durkheim, Descartes, Democritus, Plato and Kant (please forgive the temporal discord in the order in which these big names are listed here), and all the other big philosophers that Rovelli so delicately and generously reads and interprets in such a stunningly simple manner, to build his case for the illusion of the passing of time. She wishes she had the power of his mind.

She finds fucking truth in Rovelli's philosophy. She finds truth in that indeed philosophy is complicit in our illusions of the passing of time. Time rescued her in the form of the body of the black-haired woman. It was not that two hours had passed that she was therefore entitled to kindness. Rather, it was that philosophy had at once loosened its grip upon her body, in time with the hands of those twenty men on her body. She objects though, to Rovelli's suggestion that all of this is beautiful and "fair." This sounds very much like a philosopher's judgment, to her, and what we really need is a fucking judgment. What happens then, if we make fucking our way of measuring time and connecting events?

Science cannot tell her when to expect the intervention of a stranger, or a situation where arousal will happen. Science does not explain her fantasies, or the locations of her orgasms, any more than philosophy. It does not help her to understand time more and that for all this to be "fair," to find *her* sexual ethics, instead of theirs, we must let go of the instruments which come with the "fire and ice," which dupe philosophers into assuming they know all there is about fucking. Fucking is not always fair, and it is not always beautiful or beautifully painful. What is useful here is that through Rovelli, and through the many feminist and critical conceptions of non-linear time, we realize the necessity for a "fucking time." For example, asking the question as to whether we are supposed to fuck, or whether we feel that we are supposed to, when the sun is lower at the Cap, or whether another body's waiting somehow demands that we fuck, or even when our clitoris tells us we are ready. Instead, it is useful to think about what fucking tells us about time. Switching the question in this way focuses the body closely on the act of fucking: what do the orgasms she has say about the way her body needs to spend its time? This is a very different question to what time did she have her orgasm, and it is also a different question to what compelled her to act, and what was her bodily state. The latter questions simply help us to make a philosophical judgment, which as we have seen, is very unhelpful.

This, at last, is where we get to the literal and figurative heart of the matter. The next section is about kindness, and is at the heart of the new form of judgment she claims is necessary to understanding her sexual ethics. She finds that being spaceless and timeless is necessary to be kind, and to be kind is necessary to have really good sex (good is meant in both the sense of "fucking hot" sex, as well as "ethical" sex). But it is not easy and not simple, and as usual, philosophy, and philosophers, constantly obstruct her path.

To have kindness

Ethical need at the Cap is fleeting. The need (or indeed lack of need) for action is as random and/or fated as the presence and sexual interactions of certain bodies. One cannot place a temporal location on ethical need, so fucking defies time. A promise, until death do us part, is meaningless where a second is forever between two bodies who don't know how to fuck each other.

Most will have tired of the performance of fucking, that is, the "skills" that certain bodies like to show off with prowess, to name a few: I can fuck all night. I can fuck you until you can't stand up. I am hard all the time. I can do gymnastics with my tongue. The brain is the sexiest organ. I always know how to make a woman orgasm. I know where the clitoris is. I know where the g-spot is. I know a place where you can be penetrated in both your arse and your cunt. I will take you to the stars. I will fuck you like a thousand cocks. Maybe like twenty cocks. But will you fuck me like the woman with the tumbling black hair? Will you fuck me like a nurse? Will you fuck me so that forever is a second, that I can live a thousand times and never tire? Will you not take me to the dunes? Will you fuck me so softly that it's harder than I ever felt? Will you speak a new rounded language, just for me? Will you fuck me so hard that you make me feel strong, every day? Will you be kind?

We know from much research on the sex work profession across the globe that a huge part of the fucking sought by male users of sex-workers, is company, kindness and conversation.[93] We have also seen through her story that her most powerful orgasms have come from kindness, where she has felt safe, not to be protected, but to be free to her perversions without pressure to perform them and to live up to her "identity." It seems that the possibility of fucking is the generative space in which to feel what kind of sexual beings that we are. It is not her aim to make judgments or to give an analysis of sex work (this has been done far more effectively by others). What she wonders, is about what the mere presence of kindness within a sexual exchange can say about the ethics of her sexuality. It is clear that there is an appeal to kindness in sex work, between men and women, and between men and men. Indeed, the suggestion has been made many a time that sex-work is much like health work: a benevolence of non-judgmental sexuality that is succour for the soul. The most valuable of professions. But why must men pay for this erotic kindness? And what of women? Where are they to find their erotic kindness? This is what she wonders. She has sometimes found herself to be starved of the stuff, only to make protestations in the face of a denial of the very erotic power of kindness. How can this be so?

Her Philosopher: Useless biographical information won't get us anywhere.

Her: Yes, it will. I want to imagine you as you awake and everything you do in the morning, from the moment the morning drags you from sleep and you open your big brown eyes. Do you first wipe the sleep from them? Picking that small piece of yellowy grit from the corner? Isn't it fun when it's a nice big satisfying grain of sand? I expect you stretch a little. Your hair is probably stuck at all angles, like mine. I can imagine the inside of your mouth, lips slightly dry, a strong mature and spicy taste. Your skin is coated with a micro film of little pheromone bodies who have been making their home overnight among the hairs on your body. Near your arm pits they smell like they might be starting to die. I can imagine...

Her Philosopher: There's a change of intensity in your words, as you talk about my skin. Are you getting wet already? Where are you?

Her: You interrupted me. For fuck's sake, talk about an orgasm killer. But yes, I'm getting wet—it's a gentle feeling—I can feel my cunt beginning to open and my vulva is swelling. My next thought was going to be about your morning erection... where am I? I'm sitting at my writing desk. It's nearly midday and the flat is a mess. It's a day where the words are slow to come. I'm happy you called, I'm lonely. When you're not here I feel like I exist despite your absence. It's not that I want you here all the time, it's just that I feel I can just exist, not despite, not a half existence, but a whole one, when I know you will touch me later. To bear witness to your body a while, now, makes me feel less an outsider. Sometimes I'll cry in the morning, knowing you didn't choose here, this morning, this body. Talking to you reminds me that you do choose, even though you are not here. I'm wearing a mini-skirt, a scruffy T-shirt and no knickers. My skin only smells of mine, not yours. Don't you love the mixture?

Her Philosopher: I'm here now. I don't want you to cry and I don't want you to be sad. I want you to know that I think of you all the time, that even when we are apart, you are the first thing that graces my thoughts, before I brush that grit from my eyes. I want to be with you all of the time, but it is not time, yet, for that, but it will be. You don't wait for nothing, my love. I will make it so it's not waiting, that it doesn't feel like waiting, so forever feels like a second. When I wake in the morning, my first thought is you, and how the room would be filled with the smell of your...

Her: How is it true, though? Let us not kid ourselves: you wake up next to her, not me. Does that matter? Should it matter? I don't know. Sometimes, I am not jealous at all and I like that we never talk about that reality. But then I remember it and wonder if you think I don't realize that you fuck her, too. I'm not stupid you know.

Her Philosopher: Well, you are a bit stupid...

Her: It's not funny. Arsehole. Fuck off.

Her Philosopher: There is nothing, my love, nothing. You ought to know that I...

Her: You're probably lying, but it doesn't matter. It is a kind lie, a healthy one, and it makes me remember what we were talking about before. The morning. Every morning is precious with you. When I look over and see you next to me, I want to cry with joy. Do you know what I like most? I love it when you wake and urgently hug me, I can feel your cock, rock hard, pressing against my thigh and your skin is kind of cool and soft, like the first breath of air after a dreamless sleep. I like to breathe in through the sheets, they smell so intense from all of last night's fucking...

Her Philosopher: I reach around and touch your swollen pussy...

Her: Swollen from feeling your cock against my thigh, I'm wet from all the intimacy, the feeling you think of me as yours, that you can take me whenever you want, since I am in your bed. I feel your cock twitching against my thigh, desperate to be inside a woman, it drives me crazy this thought. Though if you ever describe me as your woman, or ever forced yourself on me, without me being into it, you know you can fuck right off.

Her Philosopher: Your pussy says different, you're so wet. As I reach down you turn on your back and open your legs for me, I can smell you, really strongly, I love it, your smell. I kiss you, pushing my tongue inside your mouth...

Her: I think I will come as soon as you penetrate me; my cunt always makes me think that. I would give the earth just to touch you now, or for you to come home and find me cooking for you and you wrap your arms around me...

Her Philosopher: Darling, I'm sorry, [the Philosopher's wife] has come home; I'm in my study talking to you, but I will have to go. Sweetheart, I love you and I am thinking of you and I know that you think of me too. I know it is hard and I will do everything I can to make it easier, since I know it is not fair. I will listen to your body, not with my ears, but with my nose, that's the best I can do.

Her: Be kind to both of us, that's the responsibility you have. It is impossible for either of us to do the right thing.

Her Philosopher: You won't leave me, will you?

Her: Not unless you are unkind. Not unless you tell me who I should be, or you've not had done with judgment. Not unless my body stops coming for you. Not unless my pussy stops being wet at the twitching of your cock against my thigh. Wait, no, don't do away with judgment. Your judgment about the lie you told was spot on.

Kindness can emerge in the most unlikely of places, in the most ill-advised and most unusual of relationships, and it can mean everything. Sadly, the conversation above never happened between her and her philosopher. But imagine if it did! Her point here is that a micro-kindness, a kindness that is there despite a relationship being "unusual," or "unequal," or "perverted," can mean the difference between peace and torture, orgasm or no orgasm. Kindness can bring a body to life and make it strong and able to withstand the harshest of judgments from law, from others, from oneself. This manner of kindness is about care for the sexuality of the other, and it is so unbelievably simple, yet so hard. It is hard because it means that we must rise above the law, to fuck law, in a new kind of judgment. A new kind of judgment does not care if the relationship is illicit. The truth is, though, that it takes a strong body to be kind.

If we turn to a profession that places kindness at the heart of its practice, we find a profession that is free of philosophy, yet representing the only viable and important philosophy: nursing. It is quite a cliché in some ways for her to consider nursing and fucking together, since we are all aware of the mainly male fantasy of the sexy nurse who gives him a sponge bath. In fact, there is a whole body of erotic literature and pornography dedicated to medical based fantasy.[94] We can see from Christie Watson's story that ethics for nursing (beyond the written codes of conduct) can be distilled to one notion: kindness. In Watson's story, we find true philosopher warriors whose work starts and begins with the body: attending to it from the moment it breathes (in a pile of blood and shit), and until it dies, in much the same way. The majority of nurses in the UK are women and despite having as much in the way of expertise as junior doctors, sometimes more, and just as many specialisms, they are paid a pittance and worked to the bone.[95]

The work of a sex-worker begins and ends with the body. The majority are women; some are paid a pittance and put their lives at risk on the streets, some are high class escorts and earn a very decent living. Either way, law finds it necessary (in England and Wales) to legislate sex-workers into a position that they can carry out their work, yet are in a precarious position should they ever be in danger from a client. We have seen the campaigns that sex-work is work and #decrim,[96] so that laws might change to protect sex-workers. But this will not happen, since law is terrified to talk about sex, and terrified that sex-workers might have a valued place, and moreover, that kindness might rest at the heart of our laws, rather than punishment, control and knowing.

There are problems here from her perspective. Of course, it is wonderful that a whole profession is based around not only training and hard work, but also explicit values of intuition and kindness, but how come these notions are simultaneously undermined by law, and eschewed by feminism as being "maternal" and therefore complicit in women's oppression? This is a complex and loaded area about which much has been written. What she finds important here, though, is the erotic power of simple kindness and how this ought to be available to everyone, not just those who seek out sex-workers, and those whose bodies are in trouble.

After the Cap, and after her philosopher had finally left her (before she found another), she had performed a transplant upon her sexuality. She still had filthy fantasies and she was still a bit of a whore, but she decided one important thing: when it comes to fucking, she will always be kind, in the most obvious and the most creative ways. She will not look to the law (we've seen that this does not help) instead, she will fuck by an ethic of kindness, no matter what the time, what the space, or what the body. Funny how her fucking became the best she'd ever had—it was like she'd entered the stupidly sexy world of Baker's *House of Holes*—resolutely the kindest, most sexiest fuck-story she'd ever read.

She does so aggressively, too. For the law says kindness is just for men, and just for philosophers, but no, she will have it too. The best thing about kindness is that it is infectious and it can be applied in all sorts of useful places, not only in her personal sex-life. Kindness is also a value that ethics committees ought to learn more about. Perhaps a better question, rather than: "will you be safe?", is "will you be kind?"

Fucking judgment

You look strange, without a head. It's disturbing me somewhat. Your body has all the right parts otherwise, but you have no head, just a black box. Your body still moves (albeit slowly and without direction). Your breath still quickens with my touch, and you still groan with pleasure. This will take some getting used to. I smell your chest and run my cheek gently across your hairs; it feels the same as it would with a lover who has a head. What is different, is that I can do it for as long as I like, without worrying that you will tire of me. I look at all the parts I love in a man and let my gaze linger for far longer than I would usually, you just lay there breathing. I stroke you along the length of your body, from your throat to your pubic hair, where my

hand stops. You just breathe, a slight quickening and a slight increase
in heat, your hand gently touches mine as you do. Before I get to your
cock, I suddenly freak out; this is too weird. I don't know your name!
Does it matter? I guess I can name you. I name you the name of a boy
I fancied at school. It feels better now. I touch your cock lightly, it
responds immediately and I watch it gradually grow, until the glans
glistens. You are built only for fucking, so this is your body's only
purpose. Soon your cock is thick, red, unbearably hard and leaking
with pre-orgasmic fluid. Your breath is quick and I know the lightest
touch that I give will send electric waves of pleasure through you. I
want to feel your cock against every bit of my body, it's a weird thing,
hence why I had to wait for a headless lover. I want to turn you over
and lick and smell your arsehole and spend as long as I want. There are
all kinds of micro-tastes that I have, those which don't happen in the
porn films, those which men don't understand, which aren't fetishes,
aren't "normal," they're just mine. Only a headless lover will let me
without judging and without making me into a whore, or a weirdo. A
headless lover, who is built of flesh, but no mind, Descartes's fantasy.
My pussy is dripping, this time I can spend as long as I want pressing
the head of your cock across my slit, letting it sit in the place between
my vulva and my vagina, without feeling like I have to engulf your
shaft. The only thing is, you don't have a mouth, a tongue, a voice,
eyes, hair; the developers have not managed that yet, since kindness is
difficult to program into a machine. A new kind of judgment is hard to
program into consciousness, when you only know the old kind.

She often read about sex-bots and erotic dolls with interest.
She had watched *Humans* and *Black Mirror* and frankly felt
terrified. She had also thought deeply about consent and the
ethical implications of having sex with a machine; she even
wrote a little article about it (much to the distaste of many men
who told her off for thinking such ridiculous thoughts about
machines having feelings, which is not quite her point).[97] What
she was worried about was extending a barely known human
sexual ethic toward machines. She was exhausted by the thought

of the same problems happening again, with the same vision of pleasure without kindness being programed into these new versions of ourselves. Not only could it be the case that we would be unkind to machines, but we would be unkind to ourselves again and again, by weaving the same old judgments into a new code and into a new metal.

She was also excited. Imagine if we did let go of an old kind of time, judgment and space and made proper fuckbots for everyone who wanted them![98] What about fuck-nurses? Fuck-doctors? It was looking at the philosophy of Rosi Braidotti that helped her think about inter-species and transhuman ethics. It seemed too that Braidotti was advocating the idea that we are extra careful when we deal with interspecies relations and that it is ethics, as opposed to law, that will help us decide what is right.[99] It is going to take some careful and radically open sex-talk to decide what is right in relation to sex-bots; a kind of radically open-sex talk we have not even begun when it comes to ethics, let alone laws, relating to human sexuality. The intricacies of positive (as well as negative) sexual encounters remain far too sexy and squeamish for research ethics committees, let alone the court and science labs.

As a result, addressing things like sexual violence and power-based violence in higher education and in work places has been left to radical bystander initiatives, such as Green Dot.[100] These extraordinary programs attempt to put aside the moralistic and philosophical discussions and judgments about gender and sexuality in favor of a simple, yet gentle, interventionist approach. These strategies are about "norm changing" through simply acting kindly and doing the tiniest things where someone is suffering. Having been part of the program, it is a difficult task to overcome judgment, but she can honestly say that this is the kind of strategy that might just work. The thing is, we need a parallel effort to recalibrate philosophy and sexuality (because of the experience of intervention and new judgment) and place kindness at its heart; this is much more of an effort, since it is a metaphysical change, a change in sex, in some cases a change in body, and a change in ethics, not a change in law (which is infinitely easier).

Her sexual ethics

She cannot recommend an ethical code for you, we have seen how pointless this is, from when others have tried to impose it on her. Another code would just be another judgment. In reaching an ethic, we need to understand how we fuck, to find a new way to judge, it is as simple and as complex as that. She refuses to do away with judgment since we need a judgment of some kind, or rather a sensitivity to other bodies which compels us to act one way or the other. This is a fucking judgment, rather than a legal and philosophical judgment, which tells bodies what they are, what they need and what they can have, and consequently, the sexual life that they can lead, whether they want to, or whether or not it will be orgasmic for them.

You are not sure why she did not take out my [contraceptive] coil. It's been in for longer than it should be. She knows it will be painful to remove, but that is not a good enough reason. Knowing her as you do, having gathered enough information for a judgment about her sexuality, it is, on the balance of probabilities because she wants to have more casual sex. Not having a coil in means something. Had she only desired you, then she would have taken it out as a symbol of her waiting. She would sort out her finances too, and she would stop seeing her friends so much and going out drinking and dancing until the early hours. She would certainly stop her flirting. Probably she's sleeping around, that's what these kind of women DO. After all, she was at the Cap, doing her "research." She should have signalled a deeper change, signed over her womb to you, and only you. You cannot be on the receiving end of that kind of promiscuity, that kind of lack of deed.

The kind of judgment that must stop is this kind. The ignorant kind that may not be built of malevolence, but may well be built of deep insecurity and as a result of so many centuries of silence on fucking, especially female fucking. Our fucking sexuality is beautiful, she always thought so, and we don't have to be anything we don't want to be. It is OK to be queer if you are straight, likewise it is OK to be straight if you are queer. Wherever your orgasms are, own them and move with them, let them be what compels you to act and let them be what underpins the ethics of your sexuality, rather than someone else's judgments. Think carefully about what the kindest thing to do is, to you and to other bodies (whatever kind of body they may be, whatever its history, analysis and its species), think carefully outside of philosophy (these are judgments underpinned by someone else's orgasms; why would it be helpful to you?), think carefully without your head, and in tune with your body. Read a lot, and read lots of fuck-stories to help you, don't be afraid of your tastes, think about how you want to feel: do you want to feel ill-at-ease, uncomfortable, anxious and sick and lacking in confidence, or do you want to feel just alright most of the time? Think carefully about that man (or woman, or gender-neutral body, or robot or donkey or plant) and how they make you feel, no matter how clever they say they are, or you think you are. Think and feel about what you want to keep and what you want to lose. Think with your fucking body, when and where it comes, and what this says about what and who you need in your life. Whatever you do, whoever you do, when you do it, or where, be kind.

Epilogue

[post Cap, her last message] My Philosopher, I don't want to feel tragic anymore. I don't want to feel tormented and poisonous with you haunting my dreams. I want to go out with my friends and I want to finish this PhD. I want to look at the world and feel ready for love, and not cry on my bed one more time. I want to feel not guilty when I sit and talk men, why should I? I don't want to feel your eye on me telling me I am making people do and feel things, I don't want to feel not trusted. I just want to be. I don't want to feel a punch in my stomach when I read an email or text from you. I don't want to be tormented by images of you on a family holiday. I don't want to feel like shit anymore. I want to get on and I want to have a family one day if that is what I am destined to do. I want to have a home and build a home with someone who is excited to build love with me, not to break it. I have to come to terms with the fact that it is not you and that breaks my heart and I need to mend it and allow myself to grow with all the scars that might mean. I don't want to end up frightened to love, which is how I feel now. I don't want to end up hating men, or poisonous, and at the moment, that is the way I feel it is going and I don't want that. It's a bright and sunny day today, and I am going this evening to meet my friends for dinner, and I want to do that free of this feeling now. I am boring even myself with the tragedy with which I walk. I am heartbroken, yes, but then, so what. I have lost enough time with tears and sickness, anger and frustration and loneliness and jealousy and talking about my sexuality. Enough now. I just want love now, and I hoped you would be the man, but if you can my love, let's just close this on that thought. Just That. You are my body, my heart and my blood, and you have been since I saw you sitting there at the conference when we first met. I would give everything to take back every ill-advised word, every stupid thing I have done. I can't bear the thought of life without you, but I can't do this with/without in this tone, without kindness, anymore. I just can't, my love. I am so lonely without you. That peace, that we found with each other for a while, this feeling that is so rare and so precious: I will never lose hope that this peace is out there.

Notes

1   See Chapter 3 for more details of the space specifically. In short, it is a beach where, in the summer, tens of thousands of naked people go for public sex.

2   See Paul Preciado's manifesto for a new philosophical practice, of which fucking is a crucial part: Paul Preciado (2013) *Testojunkie* (the Feminist Press, New York).

3   We might be forced to "identify" sexually in many diverse, yet ill-fitting ways, such as: male/female, heterosexual/ bisexual/homosexual/asexual/polysexual/polyamorous, vanilla, pervert, BDSM, or perhaps even victim/criminal. It may however be the case that we are many of these things in varying portions.

4   As schizophrenic and confused as our own human sexuality.

5   Academia has often been criticized as ill-equipped and often trivialising and silencing in relation to work concerning sexuality, particularly in relation to queer and female sexuality. See later in this book for more explanation, and how these problems are relevant to every-body's personal life as they "research" their sexuality.

6   Particularly in feminist thinking in relation to law and rights, vulnerability and resilience are vital human characteristics for thinking through how law ought to respond to challenges and opportunities for all bodies. See Martha Fineman and Anna Grear (eds) (2013) *Vulnerability, Reflections on a New Ethical Framework* (Ashgate, Farnham).

7   She thanks him, as promised in the Acknowledgments in that undergraduate dissertation, by continuing her work, with pride in that she is forever his student.

8   "The Dogon egg," or the "egg of the world," is a term used by Deleuze and Guattari building on the works of Marcel Griaule. The human body has within it seeds of germination

(or potentials). These seeds are not quite defined, but at the same time they are ready to grow; she found it liberating once she realized that her body, underneath its skin, could still be changed. See Gilles Deleuze and Felix Guattari, trans. Hurley, R; Seem, M and Lane, H, (2004) *Anti-Oedipus* (Continuum, London).

9 She urges you, if you haven't already, to read Michel Houellebecq (2003) *Platform* (Vintage, New York) and Michel Houellebecq (2001) *Atomised* (Vintage, New York). The figures of both Valerie and Annabelle are tragic, but within them you will see women who are bodies of troubled desire, with difficult lives, but have a powerful sexuality that is between the perhaps damaging chaste and slutty visions of femininity. His visions are challenging, but carry a truth she had never quite seen in fiction before.

10 Michel Houellebecq (2002) *Cleopâtre 2000* in Michel Houllebecq, *Lanzarote et autres textes*, Paris: Librio. See also https://hyperallergic.com/107812/the-scientific-artist-on-reading-michel-houellebecq/ accessed 13 June 2018.

11 Paul Preciado (2013) 13.

12 Ibid., 48.

13 Dianne Chisholm, "The 'Cunning Lingua' of Desire: Bodies-Language and Perverse Performativity" in Elizabeth Grosz and Elspeth Probyn (eds) (1996) *Sexy Bodies* (Routledge, Abingdon) 34.

14 Gilles Deleuze, trans. Lester, M and Stivale, C (2004) *The Logic of Sense* (Continuum, London) 338.

15 See many books on their long and passionate philosophical and bodily love-affair, for example, Elzbieta Ettinger (1994) *Hannah Arendt/Martin Heidegger* (Yale University Press, London).

16 Their anonymity is preserved, although you will find yourselves here, if you are able to listen closely enough. Thank you, though. There might be one who has managed

to fuck me back: you know who you are.

17 She was already rather enamored by his spitting and his attitude and his anarchic interpretation of Deleuzian philosophy. She even went to see him speak at the Royal Festival Hall in 2014, where she had him sign her copy of his book *Absolute Recoil* (Verso, 2014), in which he wrote: "to [She], who could have bought two packets of cigarettes instead!," before talking to her about the benefits of smoking. Come to think of it, some of this might be his fault.

18 Gilles Deleuze and Felix Guattari, trans. Hurley, R, Seem, M and Lane, H, (2004) *Anti-Oedipus* (Continuum, London), 325: "microscopic transsexuality, resulting in the woman containing as many men as the man, and the man as many women, all capable of entering—men with women, women with men—into relations of production of desire that overturn the statistical order of the sexes. Making love is not just becoming as one, or even two, but becoming as a hundred thousand. Desiring-machines or the nonhuman sex: not one or even two sexes, but *n* sexes."

19 Gretchen Riordan, "Haemosexuality," in Frida Beckman (ed) (2011) *Deleuze and Sex* (Edinburgh University Press, Edinburgh), 87.

20 Ronald Bogue, "Alien Sex," in Frida Beckman (ed) (2011) *Deleuze and Sex* (Edinburgh University Press, Edinburgh) 47.

21 Valerie De Craene (2017) "Fucking Geographers! Or the epistemological consequences of neglecting the lusty researcher's body," *Gender Place and Culture*, 2017, 24:3, 449-464.

22 Gregg Lambert, *Who's Afraid of Deleuze and Guattari?* (Continuum, 2006) 149.

23 Authors such as Elizabeth Grosz are heavy-weight presences in creating the theoretical anti-Cartesian conditions

for the mere possibility of this resistance too, through the revolutionary re-situation of the feminine body as disruptive of traditional understandings of the body, space and time, as well as sexuality: see Elizabeth Grosz (1994) *Volatile Bodies* (Indiana University Press, Indianapolis) and in particular, Elizabeth Grosz (1995) *Space, Time and Perversion* (Routledge, London).

24   Looking at Eric Berkowitz (2012) *Sex and Punishment: Four Thousand Years of Judging Desire* (Counterpoint, Berkeley) we can see that law has become more generous in its judgment and punishment of sexual encounters. No longer, for example, would one be punished so severely (by death on occasion) for adultery. However, in the recent English legal case of R v McNally [2013] EWCA Crim 1051, the law revealed its "transphobic" tendencies and decides that deception as to gender, over and above factors such as age, marital status, wealth and HIV status, is a valid factor that will vitiate consent (paras. 23-27 of the judgment). This manages to simultaneously embed gender categories, as well as privilege gender as a universal concern within sexual encounters (above such concerns as wealth, age, attractiveness and so on).

25   In the criminal justice system, there are consistent efforts by academics and lawyers alike to adapt the rules of evidence to ensure that the law's processes avoid allowing juries and judges to make assumptions about victim behaviors in sexual offences, and how a victim "ought" to behave. See for example Louise Ellinson (2005) "Closing the Credibility Gap: the prosecutorial use of expert witness testimony in sexual assault cases," *International Journal of Evidence and Proof*, 9, 239-268. The "offender" identity can lead also to unjust assumptions too, just as the "victim" identity. Any identity can misrepresent anybody.

26   See, for example: https://www.theguardian.com/commen

tisfree/2018/feb/04/metoophd-reveals-shocking-examples-of-academic-sexism; https://www.theguardian.com/higher-education-network/2017/dec/01/as-a-young-academic-i-was-repeatedly-sexually-harassed-at-conferences and http s://jezebel.com/academias-shitty-men-list-has-around-2-000-entries-deta-1821991028 all accessed on 13 June 2018, to name only a few and the very early stages of the realization of sexual harassment in academia.

27 See David Bell, "Fucking Geography, Again" in Browne, K et al (eds) (2009) *Geographies of Sexualities: Theory Practices and Politics* (Surrey, Ashgate).

28 See Victoria Brooks (2018) "Fucking Law (A New Methodological Movement)" in *Journal of Organizational Ethnography*, 7:1, 31-43 for an examination of the power of the word "fuck" in academia, and in relation to the need to censor so-called profane sex-talk.

29 Paul Preciado (2013) 42.

30 See Gilles Deleuze trans. Hurley, R., (1988) *Spinoza Practical Philosophy* (City Light Books, San Francisco) 127 and note below.

31 See Andreas Philippopoulos-Mihalopoulos (2015) *Spatial Justice: Body, Lawscape, Atmosphere* (Routledge, London) 206. Conatus is a term used by the philosopher, Benedict de Spinoza and by Gilles Deleuze. For Spinoza conatus was a key idea for understanding the way the body moves and can be understood as "perseverance" and "striving." In Deleuzian philosophy this became desire, with all its possibilities for sexuality, movement and transformation. For Philippopoulos-Mihalopoulos conatus means that bodies are entitled to rights, but rights that the body can claim as fitting, "rules of living" not as those decided for it based on judgments by the court.

32 Paul Preciado (2013) 391.

33 Ibid at 424.

34 Jamie Murray (2013) *Emergent Law* (Routledge, London) 11.

35 See Luis De Miranda, L (2013) "Is a New Life Possible: Deleuze and the Lines," *Deleuze Studies*, 7:1, 106-152, 108.

36 Idem.

37 See the development of the concept in a famous lecture given by Foucault: Michel Foucault, trans. Miskowiec, J (1986) "Of Other Spaces: Utopias and Heterotopias," *Diacritics*, 16:1, 22-27, and a modern application of this to a beach of "deviance" albeit in the context of homosexual cruising, Andriotis, K (2010) "Heterotopic Erotic Oases: The Public Nude Beach Experience," *Annals of Tourism Research*, 37:4, 1076-1096.

38 See Houngbedji, A and Guillem, E (2015) "Profiles and sexual practices of current and past swingers interviewed on French websites," *Sexologies*, 25:1, 1-4 for a comprehensive statistical analysis of the gender dynamic in swinging practices. Although the methodological approach in this piece is rigorous, and includes empirical data relating to experiences on swinging "dating" sites, it provides little in the way of personal insight. See also Kimberley, C and Hans, J (2015) "From Fantasy to Reality: A Grounded Theory of Experiences in the Swinging Lifestyle," *Archives of Sexual Behaviour*, DOI:10.1007/s10508-015-0621-2. Here the authors undertake structured interviews to obtain insights into "marital satisfaction." At the Cap, at that time, she guesses she was outnumbered certainly more than 10:1 by single men, and by an even greater ratio in relation to male/female couples.

39 Chris Ashford (2012) "Heterosexuality, Public Places and Policing" in Johnson, P and Dalton, D *Policing Sex* (Routledge, London) 44-45.

40 Ibid at 51.

41 Idem.

42 Idem.

43   Thank you, Jon Binnie, who examined her PhD. His love for her work on that day inspires her every day.

44   Jon Binnie, "The Erotic Possibilities of the City" in Bell, D et al (2001) *Pleasure Zones* (New York, Syracuse University Press) 107.

45   Ibid at 108.

46   Seideman, S (1994) "Queer-ing Sociology. Socializing Queer Theory: An Introduction" as cited by Les Moran "The Public Sex of the Judiciary: the appearance of the irrelevant and the invisible," in Jones, J et al (eds) (2012) *Gender, Sexualities and Law* (Routledge, London) 81.

47   Idem.

48   See Gilles Deleuze, trans. Boyman, A, (2001) *Pure Immanence: Essays on a Life* (Zone Books, New York). Deleuze gives an example of ethics in practice, where a dying Dickensian rogue is found by people who hold him in contempt. Despite their feelings of revilement, those who find him experience an eagerness for the slightest signs of life. As he returns to life however, they again turn mean and crude toward him. In this moment of death being immanent within life, a personal/impersonal moment emerges where all worlds meet to do what is best to make the rogue's body stronger. This moment transcends the hatred they feel since personal consciousness dissolves into the encounter.

49   Francois Laruelle, trans. Gangle, R, (2010) *Philosophies of Difference* (Continuum, London) 210.

50   Ray Brassier (2007) *Nihil Unbound* (Palgrave Macmillan, London) 119.

51   See Hickman, C (2015) "François Laruelle: Future Struggle, Gnosis and the last Humaneity" retrieved from http://non. copyriot.com/francois-laruelle-future-struggle-gnosis-and-the-last-humaneity/.

52   Idem.

53   Extract from field notes, 15 July 2014, 6:20 a.m.: "This sand

of 100,000 orgasms, just allowing me to sit, and how I desire just one of those at the hands of just one man, such a curious thing."

54   Valerie De Craene (2017).

55   Tim Dean (2009) *Unlimited Intimacy: Reflections on the Subculture of Barebacking* (University of Chicago Press, Chicago) 8.

56   Valerie De Craene (2017).

57   Alexander Lambevski (2001) "The flesh of gay sex and the surprise of affect," *International Journal of Critical Psychology*, 3, 29-48, 1-2.

58   Ibid. at p2.

59   Gavin Brown (2008) "Ceramics, clothing and other bodies: affective geographies of homoerotic cruising encounters," *Social and Cultural Geography*, 9:8, 915-932.

60   Jon Binnie (2004) "The Globalization of Sexuality" as cited by Gavin Brown (2008) 915.

61   Gavin Brown (2008) 917.

62   Eileen Honan (2007) "Writing a Rhizome: An (im)plausible Methodology," *International Journal of Qualitative Studies in Education*, 20:5, 531-546, 535.

63   Brooke Hofsess and Jennifer Sonenberg (2013) "Enter: Ho/rhizoanalysis," *Cultural Studies*, 20:10, 1-10, 1.

64   Idem.

65   See Alexander Wendt (2015) *Quantum Mind and Social Science* (Cambridge University Press, Cambridge) 47: "Prior to its measurement, the wave function constitutes a complete description of a quantum system; there is no definite reality hiding behind the wave function about which we could obtain further knowledge if only we had the means."

66   Retrieved from http://location-mer-capdagde.wifeo.com/la-residence.php accessed on 13 June 2018.

67   Retrieved from http://www.capdagdefrance.co.uk/maps/ accessed on 13 June 2018.

68 This view can be retrieved from Google Maps (Street View) at https://www.google.co.uk/maps/@43.2957336,3.5262069, 3a,75y,90h,89.44t/data=!3m6!1e1!3m4!1s--ysoiZTVltR8_13tf N8UA!2e0!7i13312!8i6656 accessed on 13 June 2018.

69 Fabio D'Orlando (2010) "Swinger Economics," Working Paper, Dipartimento di Scienze Economiche Università di Cassino, 1/2010.

70 See Harp, S (2011) "Demanding Vacation au naturel: European Nudism and Postwar Municipal Development on the French Riviera," *Journal of Modern History*, 83:3, 513-543 for an in-depth analysis of the historical and economic development of the Cap.

71 Fabio D'Orlando (2010) 298.

72 Trachman, M (2012) "The Pornographers Trade: A discredited professional group's rhetoric," *control and know-how*, 54:1.

73 Ross Velton (2003) *The Naked Truth about Cap d'Agde* (Scarlett, Oh!, California) 80-81.

74 Idem.

75 Serena D'Onofrio (2011) "Bisexuality, Gaia, Eros: Portals to the Arts of Loving," *Journal of Bisexuality*, 11:2-3, 176-194, 187.

76 Idem.

77 Idem.

78 See Nicholson Baker (2011) *House of Holes* (Simon & Schuster, London); Nicholson Baker (1993) *Vox* (Vintage, New York); Nicholson Baker (1994) *Fermata* (Vintage, New York).

79 Nicholson Baker (2011) 56.

80 Charlotte Roche (2009) *Wetlands* (Fourth Estate, London) 21.

81 Deleuze and Guattari found the orgasm to be "deplorable" since it serves to connect pleasure with lack. The pursuit of pleasure is thus always tied to the site of orgasm, which then produces your sexual identity. Post-Deleuzian thought has sought to reframe orgasm as positivity and untie pleasures

from a capitalist-appropriated desire. See Beckman, F (ed) (2011).

82 See Helen Hester (2018) *Xenofeminism* (Polity Press, Cambridge).

83 See Chapter 6. If we are to move with the spirit of Hester's interruption through the technological movement of Xenofeminism (supra), we must give careful thought to how we are extending our barely understood all-too-human sexual ethic to sex-robots.

84 Deleuze, G (1997).

85 Idem: "It is the dream that makes the lots turn (Ezekiel's wheel) and makes the forms pass in procession. In the dream, judgments are hurled into the void, without encountering the resistance of a milieu that would subject them to the exigencies of knowledge or experience; therefore, the question of judgment is first knowing whether one is dreaming or not."

86 Idem: "Whenever we turn away from judgment toward justice, we enter into a dreamless sleep."

87 See Newton, E (1993) "My Best Informant's Dress: The Erotic Equation in Fieldwork," *Cultural Anthropology*, 8, 3-23.

88 See https://www.theguardian.com/world/2018/apr/25/raw-hatred-why-incel-movement-targets-terrorises-women; https://www.independent.co.uk/news/long_reads/incel-what-is-involuntary-celibates-elliot-rodger-alek-minassian-canada-terrorism-a8335816.html ; and https://incels.me/ accessed on 13 June 2018, if you are feeling brave.

89 Laurent de Sutter (2017) *Narcocapitalism* (Polity Press).

90 Idem.

91 Carlo Rovelli (2018) *The Order of Time* (Allen Lane, London).

92 Ibid., at 182.

93 See https://en.wikipedia.org/wiki/Girlfriend_experience accessed on 13 June 2018.

94 See here for an explanation https://en.wikipedia.org/wiki/ Medical_fetishism accessed on 13 June 2018, and limitless erotic stories and videos.

95 Christie Watson (2018) *The Language of Kindness: A Nurse's Story* (Chatto and Windus, London).

96 See https://twitter.com/hashtag/decrim?lang=en accessed on 13 June 2018.

97 See Victoria Brooks (2018) "Samantha's Suffering: why sex machines should have rights too" at https://theconversation. com/samanthas-suffering-why-sex-machines-should-have-rights-too-93964 accessed on 13 June 2018.

98 See https://www.cnet.com/news/abyss-creations-ai-sex-ro bots-headed-to-your-bed-and-heart/ accessed on 13 June 2018, in relation to how sex-bots could address loneliness. The question remains open as to how though, and for whom.

99 Idem.

100 See https://en.wikipedia.org/wiki/Green_Dot_Bystander_ Intervention and https://alteristic.org/ accessed on 13 June 2018, for more details.

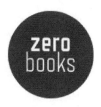

CULTURE, SOCIETY & POLITICS

Contemporary culture has eliminated the concept and public
figure of the intellectual. A cretinous anti-intellectualism
presides, cheer-led by hacks in the pay of multinational
corporations who reassure their bored readers that there is no
need to rouse themselves from their stupor. Zer0 Books knows
that another kind of discourse – intellectual without being
academic, popular without being populist – is not only possible:
it is already flourishing. Zer0 is convinced that in the unthinking,
blandly consensual culture in which we live, critical and engaged
theoretical reflection is more important than ever before.
If you have enjoyed this book, why not tell other readers by
posting a review on your preferred book site.

Recent bestsellers from Zero Books are:

In the Dust of This Planet
Horror of Philosophy vol. 1
Eugene Thacker
In the first of a series of three books on the Horror of Philosophy,
In the Dust of This Planet offers the genre of horror as a way of
thinking about the unthinkable.
Paperback: 978-1-84694-676-9 ebook: 978-1-78099-010-1

Capitalist Realism
Is there no alternative?
Mark Fisher
An analysis of the ways in which capitalism has presented itself
as the only realistic political-economic system.
Paperback: 978-1-84694-317-1 ebook: 978-1-78099-734-6

Rebel Rebel
Chris O'Leary
David Bowie: every single song. Everything you want to know,
everything you didn't know.
Paperback: 978-1-78099-244-0 ebook: 978-1-78099-713-1

Cartographies of the Absolute
Alberto Toscano, Jeff Kinkle
An aesthetics of the economy for the twenty-first century.
Paperback: 978-1-78099-275-4 ebook: 978-1-78279-973-3

Malign Velocities
Accelerationism and Capitalism
Benjamin Noys
Long listed for the Bread and Roses Prize 2015, *Malign Velocities* argues against the need for speed, tracking acceleration as the symptom of the ongoing crises of capitalism.
Paperback: 978-1-78279-300-7 ebook: 978-1-78279-299-4

Meat Market
Female Flesh under Capitalism
Laurie Penny
A feminist dissection of women's bodies as the fleshy fulcrum of capitalist cannibalism, whereby women are both consumers and consumed.
Paperback: 978-1-84694-521-2 ebook: 978-1-84694-782-7

Poor but Sexy
Culture Clashes in Europe East and West
Agata Pyzik
How the East stayed East and the West stayed West.
Paperback: 978-1-78099-394-2 ebook: 978-1-78099-395-9

Romeo and Juliet in Palestine
Teaching Under Occupation
Tom Sperlinger
Life in the West Bank, the nature of pedagogy and the role of a university under occupation.
Paperback: 978-1-78279-637-4 ebook: 978-1-78279-636-7

Sweetening the Pill
or How We Got Hooked on Hormonal Birth Control
Holly Grigg-Spall
Has contraception liberated or oppressed women? *Sweetening the Pill* breaks the silence on the dark side of hormonal contraception.
Paperback: 978-1-78099-607-3 ebook: 978-1-78099-608-0

Why Are We The Good Guys?
Reclaiming your Mind from the Delusions of Propaganda
David Cromwell
A provocative challenge to the standard ideology that Western power is a benevolent force in the world.
Paperback: 978-1-78099-365-2 ebook: 978-1-78099-366-9

Printed and bound by PG in the USA

USA2019PGIL